D1236678

INFORMATION
RESOURCES IN TOXICOLOGY

INFORMATION RESOURCES IN TOXICOLOGY

Philip Wexler

Elsevier Biomedical
New York • Amsterdam • Oxford

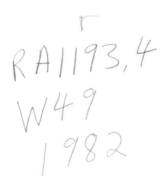

Elsevier Science Publishing Co., Inc.
52 Vanderbilt Avenue, New York, New York 10017

Sole distributors outside the USA and Canada:
Elsevier Science Publishers B.V.
P.O. Box 211, 1000 AE Amsterdam, The Netherlands

Library of Congress Cataloging in Publication Data

Wexler, Philip.
    Information resources in toxicology.

    Includes index.
    1. Toxicology—Information services—United States. 2. Toxicology—
    Bibliography. 3. Toxicology—United States—Societies, etc. I.
    Title [DNLM: 1. Toxicology—Bibliography. 2. Toxicology—
    Directories. ZQV 600 W454i]
RA1193.4.W49   616.9'007   81-9734
ISBN 0-444-00616-8   AACR2

Manufactured in the United States of America

And even in our times it is said, venomous animals poison the water after the setting of the sun, so that the good animals cannot drink of it, but in the morning after the sunrise, comes the unicorn and dips his horn into the stream driving away the poison from it . . . this I have seen for myself.

—John of Hesse

To Prinz

Contents

Preface

Although literature in toxicology is proliferating at a phenomenal rate, and access to this literature by use of computer data bases and other tools is fairly adequate, there has as yet been no succinct guide directing devotees of toxicology to the major sources of information in the field. This guide is an attempt to fill this void. It is a selective and annotated list of information resources. I have tried to select material that is or has the potential of being widely and frequently used and is exceptional in its content and presentation. In addition, I have included material that may not necessarily be of reference use but that is representative of a subject or format. Both relatively broad areas of toxicology and more specific fields of interest have been covered.

Toxicology deals with chemical, physical, and biological (i.e., plant and animal toxins) hazards to man. Chemicals have unavoidably been emphasized. The large number of potentially dangerous commercial chemicals and the large populations exposed to them has resulted in a focus of attention on chemical hazards in research, regulations, and press coverage. I have tried to balance this emphasis by including substantial resources on physical and biological hazards.

For the purposes of this guide, the following areas arc within the scope of toxicology: industrial and household chemicals and substances, food, drugs, cosmetics, gases, radiation and radioactive substances, sound, heat, light, laser, microwave, metals, minerals, trace elements, biotoxins (mushrooms, plants, insect stings, snake and marine life venoms), environmental pollutants, pesticides, industrial hygiene and occupational medicine, analytical techniques, chemical and forensic toxicology, epidemiology, contamination of water and air, carcinogenesis, mutagenesis, teratogenesis and reproductive toxicology, behavioral toxicology, toxicity testing, legislation, regulations, and societal issues, veterinary toxicology, and target systems toxicology. The concentration is that of health effects. Therefore, topics such as management and storage of wastes and waste disposal; engineering, equipment, and monitoring aspects; mechanical aspects of pollution, and ecology and environmental impact where man is not considered a key component of the biosphere are peripheral to the scope of this guide. In addition, the following topics have not been emphasized: alcohol and tobacco, drug abuse, allergy and hypersensitivity, and mechanical and traffic hazards.

The materials chosen are in English and the organizations are primarily within the United States. One chapter provides a glimpse into international activities.

The chapter divisions devised for this guide are somewhat arbitrary, although not indiscriminate. Some of the materials in both the periodicals and books sections, for instance, could have been merged into a chapter on handbooks (e.g., RTECS, TOSCA Inventory, etc.). Then, the associated problem of how to categorize items that were partially handbooks of data and partially expository prose, would have arisen. Directories, on the other hand, for which there is a separate chapter, could have been dispersed among the serials and books. After much thought, I have settled on the organization that follows.

The guide has been organized in a manner that should be most convenient for scanning as well as for accessing a particular item or class of items. The overall organization, along with the indexes, should provide sufficient access. I have avoided creating too many categories and chapters as this tends to confound matters and create an extremely disjointed product in a field where there is great overlap in subdisciplines.

There was a great temptation to make this guide much larger than it is, since there is no shortage of material. This, however, would have become unwieldy and defeated the purpose of providing a core list of the most necessary and useful information.

All quoted passages within the annotations are taken from the item cited—for serials this information usually appears as scope notes or information for authors; for books, the quoted sections have usually been extracted from the preface.

This guide was compiled with the assistance of many individuals and organizations. Holdings lists of libraries, individual specialists' recommendations, reading lists for classes in toxicology, compilations of materials used in the creation of data bases, and library card catalogs were all consulted. The outstanding facilities of the National Library of Medicine, the Library of Congress, the National Institutes of Health Library, as well as those of other Washington area libraries, were utilized to examine virtually all of the items.

Special thanks are owed to the following individuals who provided valuable guidance and support throughout this project: Arthur Wykes, Mel Spann, Aurora K. Reich, Pat O'Brien, and Sally Moulton.

Since a guide such as this quickly becomes outdated it is essential that revised editions be published periodically. Comments and suggestions from readers regarding the content and organization of the guide as it exists, items omitted, those that seem unnecessary, or alternate ways of presenting the material would be greatly appreciated, as they will result in future editions of even greater value to the toxicologist.

The views expressed in this book are the personal opinions of the author and should not be taken to represent the views of any organization with which he is or has been associated.

Philip Wexler

INFORMATION
RESOURCES IN TOXICOLOGY

PART I

REFERENCE SOURCES

Chapter 1

Historical Perspective

Any guide to toxicology resources would be incomplete without at least a brief account of the field's early history and mention of some significant contributors to its scientific evolution. Toxic effects of various natural and synthetic agents have been observed through the ages. Similarly, there have been continuous investigations of mechanisms of action of poisons and a search for remedies.

Poisons have a long, if less than honorable, tradition in subduing animals and man. Socrates is just one example of state execution by poison (via hemlock).

Some of the major accomplishments of early toxicology were related to the recognition of the connection between work and disease. Agricola, Paracelsus, and Ramazzini all linked aspects of selected occupations to ailments from which workers in these professions suffered. Percival Pott's observation that chimney sweeps in 18th Century England suffered from a higher than expected incidence of scrotal cancer is a landmark in occupational disease, carcinogenesis, and epidemiology.

The few items listed in this section chronologically are not meant to trace the history of toxicology (a monumental project in itself and well worth the efforts of someone capable of such a task), but to give a sense of perspective to the remainder of the book and to aquaint the reader with some key personalities.

1. *Papyrus Ebers*. Translated by B. Ebbell. Copenhagen. Munksgaard. 1937.

> This ancient Egyptian medical document outlines remedies for assorted disease states. The remedy for bites by men is a mixture of frankincense, yellow ochre, and gall of goat. Another useful "remedy to expel stinking in the summer" consists of frankincense, pignon, and myrrh. One of the earliest pharmacopeias in existence.

2. Nicander. *The Poems and Poetical Fragments.* Cambridge. University Press. 1953.

   Ancient Greece. Nicander is responsible for two documents (*Therica* and *Alexipharmaca*), both written in poetical form, concerned with toxicology. The *Therica* covers venoms and stings of snakes, spiders, scorpions, insects, lizards, fish and their remedies. The *Alexipharmaca* describes additional toxins (e.g., aconite, blister beetles, hemlock, etc.), their effects, and treatments.

3. Agricola G. *De Re Metallica* (translated from the first Latin edition of 1556). London. The Mining Magazine, Salisbury House. 1912.

   At the time of its publication, this was the most exhaustive textbook on mining and metallurgy, as well as on the workers in these fields, that had ever been created. Agricola devotes a small but significant portion of his text to health effects and ailments of miners (see Book VI). Agricola begins this brief section with, "It remains for me to speak of the ailments and accidents of miners, and of the methods by which they can guard against these, for we should always devote more care to maintaining our health, that we may freely perform our bodily functions, than to making profits. Of the illnesses, some affect the joints, others attack the lungs, some the eyes, and finally some are fatal to men." The author also describes various demons, which he refers to as "pernicious pests," that inhabit the mines.

4. Orfila MP. *A General System of Toxicology or, a Treatise on Poisons, Found in the Mineral, Vegetable, and Animal Kingdoms, Considered in their Relations with Physiology, Pathology, and Medical Jurisprudence* (a translation from the French). Philadelphia. M. Carey & Son. 1817.

   One of the earliest comprehensive treatises on poisons. A sort of forerunner to Arena. Orfila's book is intended to guide the practitioner in diagnosing and treating poisonings. The book is arranged by class of poison—the corrosive, the astringent, the acrid, and the narcotic. Poisons are precisely described in terms of physical and chemical properties, actions, and treatments. Numerous experimental and case studies are described. This is a highly systematic and fascinating guide to poisoning. For instance, Orfila divides up the possible cases of poisoning by verdegris that may present themselves to the practitioner: "First Case: The Patient is living: the rest of the Poison can be examined. Second Case: The Patient is living: the whole of the Poison has been swallowed: the Matter vomited may be examined. Third Case: The Patient is living: the whole of the Poison has been swallowed: the Vomitings cannot be procured. Fourth Case: The Patient is Dead." Note—Dr. Orfila's text under the third case is, "Chemistry cannot enable us to throw any light on this difficult and embarrassing case." Orfila cites the work of many other physicians and is generous in giving credit.

5. Orfila MP. *Directions for the Treatment of Persons Who Have Taken Poison, and Those in a State of Apparent Death; Together with the Means of Detecting Poisons and Adulterations in Wine; Also, of Distinguishing Real from Apparent Death* (a translation from the French). Baltimore. Nathaniel G. Maxwell. 1819.

This is a practical but much briefer guide to poisonings than the aforementioned treatise. Properties of poisons have been kept to a minimum. Experiments and cases have been eliminated. The concentration is on effects and treatment. The text is very much to the point and must have been a handy tool for physicians 200 years ago. Orfila recognized the hazards of lead on painters. A distillation of toxicological wisdom.

6. Thompson CJS. *Poisons and Poisoners*. London. Harold Shaylor. 1931.

An entertaining historical survey of poisons used for criminal purposes. The author begins with poisons used by primitive man and ancient civilizations. Some of the fascinating topics covered are women poisoners, the Italian School of Poisoners, a professional poisoner and his fees, love-philters, poison plots and conspiracies, etc. Many poison trials and mysteries, the famous and the less well known, are covered. Illustrated.

7. Paracelsus. *Von der Bergsucht und anderen Bergkrankheiten* (1567). (On the Miners' Sickness and Other Diseases of Miners) in *Four Treatises of Theophrastus von Hohenheim called Paracelsus*. Baltimore. Johns Hopkins Press. 1941.

Whereas Agricola devotes a small portion of De Re Metallica to diseases of the mines, Paracelsus' entire treatise is concerned with miners' sickness, particularly pulmonary ailments. A fascinating mixture of science, philosophy, and mysticism. Poisonous minerals and other chemicals and their fumes are discussed. Particular attention is paid to mercury and its aerial spirits (often referred to as "spiritus") and their action on the lungs. Paracelsus is perhaps most famous for recognizing that "All substances are poisons; there is none which is not a poison. The right dose differentiates a poison and a remedy." Paracelsus was quite aware of the distinction between acute and chronic toxicity as when he says, "If arsenic is ingested there is a rapid sudden death; if however the body is not taken, but its spiritus, the latter makes a year out of an hour, i.e. whatever the body accomplishes in ten hours, the spiritus does in ten years. Also there does not occur as terrible a death as when the body itself is present." Very rewarding reading for anyone interested in the ideas of a truly key figure in toxicology.

8. Ramazzini B. *De Morbis Artificum Dintriba* (Modena, 1700). *Diseases of Workers* (English Translation). New York. Hafner. (part of the History of

Medicine Series issued under the auspices of the library of the New York Academy of Medicine). 1964.

Ramazzini is considered the father of occupational medicine. He was the first to recommend that, in addition to questions to be asked of a patient as recommended by Hippocrates, the physician should ask an additional question: "What occupation does he follow?" Among the work groups discussed are miners of metal, gilders, chemists, tinsmiths, painters, blacksmiths, tobacco workers, vintners, salt makers, sedentary workers, farmers, soap makers, etc. An admirable early treatise on the hazards of occupations.

9. Pott P. *Cancer Scroti* in *Chirurgical Observations Relative to the Cataract, the Polypus of the Nose, the Cancer of the Scrotum, the Different Kinds of Ruptures, and the Mortification of the Toes and Feet*. London. Hawes, Clark, and Collins. 1775.

Pott links the occupation of chimney sweeps with cancer of the scrotum. ". . . every body is acquainted with the disorders to which painters, plummers, glaziers, and the workers in white lead, are liable; but there is a disease as peculiar to a certain set of people which has not, at least to my knowledge, been publickly noticed; I mean the chimney-sweepers' cancer."

Chapter 2

Books

The books represent a varied selection of textbooks, reference works, handbooks, proceedings, government reports, etc. A few items are individual volumes of monographic series, listed because the topic is not adequately represented elsewhere or because it is an exceptionally noteworthy treatment of the subject.

Books have been chosen that are generally thorough, well documented, useful for reference, and widely used or deserving of wide usage. The books cover fairly broad areas of toxicology with occasional exceptions for narrower topics of special interest and importance. Most of the books listed have been published since 1975 and new books in toxicology are being published at a high rate.

Perhaps the greatest difficulty was in dividing the books into logical, coherent categories. There is a great deal of overlap within the subfields of toxicology. It is hoped that the classification selected will prove useful. "See also" references will lead the reader from one category to related books in another category. These cross references should not be used exclusively because there are many more intricate connections too fine in detail to cite. The combination of "see also" references, general scanning of titles and annotations, and the use of the index should provide adequate access to the books listed.

The broad areas chosen for the books are as follows:

1. General Textbooks
2. Analytical Toxicology
3. Biotoxins (Plant or Animal)
4. Carcinogenesis, Mutagenesis, Teratogenesis
5. Clinical Toxicology (includes Forensic Toxicology)
6. Cosmetics
7. Drugs

8. Environmental Toxicology (i.e., hazards of environmental substances not covered in any other category)
9. Food
10. Legislation, Regulations, and Societal Issues
11. Metals
12. Occupational Health and Industrial Hygiene
13. Pesticides
14. Physical Hazards (including Radiation, Noise)
15. Target Systems (e.g., Eye, Skin, Blood, etc.)
16. Veterinary Toxicology
17. Miscellaneous

General Textbooks

10. Ariens EJ, Simonis AM. *Introduction to General Toxicology,* revised printing. New York. Academic Press. 1978.

> A concise textbook offering a general introduction to the field. Useful as an overview of toxicology. A new chapter in the revised printing covers environmental toxicology.

11. Doull J, Klaasen CD, Amdur MO, eds. *Casarett and Doull's Toxicology,* 2nd ed. New York. Macmillan. 1980.

> Perhaps the most widely used text and overall reference work in the broad field of toxicology. Separated into five sections: general principles, systemic, toxic agents, environmental, and applications. New chapters added to the second edition are "Genetic Toxicology," "Water and Soil Pollutants," and "Regulatory Toxicology." Extensive, updated references and supplemental readings. Inside and outside the classroom, Casarett and Doull is always a fine source for background and orientation.

12. Guthrie, FE, Perry JJ, eds. *Introduction to Environmental Toxicology.* New York. Elsevier. 1980.

> Intended as a textbook for the advanced undergraduate and graduate student. 35 chapters on energy, nuclear power, aquatic toxicology, oil in the biosphere, food additives, regulation, etc. Includes case histories of pollution incidents and effects, e.g., PCBs and the Hudson River, Cincinnati and air pollution. Suggested readings follow each chapter.

13. Hodgson E, Guthrie FE, eds. *Introduction to Biochemical Toxicology.* New York. Elsevier. 1980.

> A basic text in toxicology for the undergraduate or graduate student. In 22 separately authored chapters this book sets the groundwork for advanced study. Topics such as toxicokinetics, metabolism, elimination, mutagenesis and carcinogenesis, hepatotoxicity, and natural toxins are

covered. There are chapters, as well, on chronic testing and short term tests. Suggested readings follow each chapter. With toxicology usually relegated to a position subservient to and included within pharmacology, it is refreshing to hear the editors argue that ''it may be more appropriate to consider pharmacology a branch of toxicology.''

14. Loomis TA. *Essentials of Toxicology*. Philadelphia. Lea and Febiger. 1978.

   A slim, basic text offering a concise introduction to the field.

15. Purdom PW, ed. *Environmental Health,* 2nd ed. New York. Academic Press. 1980.

   A textbook on the health effects of the environment on man. Provides an overview of problems of infectious diseases, foods, water, air, solid waste, radiation, industrial hygiene, housing, noise, accident prevention, environmental planning, etc.

Analytical Toxicology

16. Getz ME. *Paper and Thin Layer Chromatographic Analysis of Environmental Toxicants*. London. Heyden. 1980.

   Using simple chromatographic techniques, environmental toxicants may be monitored. Assays are described for drugs, animal feed additives, air and water pollutants, pesticides, food additives, cosmetics, and naturally occurring toxicants. One chapter describes chromatographic techniques and reagents in general.

17. Sunshine I, ed. *Handbook of Analytical Toxicology*. Cleveland. Chemical Rubber Company. 1969.

   ''In addition to collating the physical and chemical properties of drugs and chemical hazards, summaries of published methods for their detection in biological specimens are presented.''

18. Sunshine I, ed. *Methodology for Analytical Toxicology*. Cleveland. CRC Press. 1975.

   Enables the chemist to determine analysis of drugs in biological fluids as an aid to the physician in order to decide whether poisoning has occurred. Industrial toxicology and occupational hazards are not within the scope of this book.

19. Thoma JJ, Bondo PB, Sunshine I. *Guidelines for Analytical Toxicology Programs,* 2 volumes. Cleveland CRC Press. 1977.

   ''Intended to provide practical guidelines to physicians and laboratory directors who are anticipating development of a toxicology service, and to those whose programs are underway but who wish to expand their services ... Useful to the laboratory technologist who must use the many different isolation and identification techniques peculiar to the field."

See also:

Bowman MC. *Carcinogens and Related Substances: Analytical Chemistry for Toxicology.* [under *Carcinogenesis, Mutagenesis, Teratogenesis*]

Biotoxins

20. Bettini S. *Arthropod Venoms.* Berlin. Springer-Verlag. 1978.

Volume 48 of the *Handbook of Experimental Pharmacology.* In 25 chapters, specialists discuss chemistry, pharmacology, mechanism of action, and toxicology of arthropod venoms.

21. Bucherl W, Buckley EE, Devlofeu V. *Venomous Animals and Their Venoms,* 3 volumes. New York. Academic Press. 1968-1971.

Covers vertebrates and invertebrates. Concentrates on snakes. Also chapters on insects, saurians, battrachians, fish, centipedes, spiders, scorpions, mollusks, coelenterates, echinoderms, and anelids.

22. Eaker D, Wadstrom T, eds. *Natural Toxins.* Oxford. Pergamon Press 1980.

Contains 83 of the papers presented at the 6th International Symposium on Animal, Plant and Microbial Toxins held at Uppsala, Sweden in 1979. These are primarily review in nature. Topics include envenomation pathophysiology, the immune system, effects of blood coagulation and fibrinolysis, cytolytic toxins, phospholipases, enterotoxins, lipid A and endotoxin, edema producing toxin, toxins with intracellular targets, polypeptide neurotoxins, neurotransmitter release and venom toxins, botilinum and tetanus toxins.

23. Halstead BW, Halstead LG, eds. *Poisonous and Venomous Marine Animals of the World.* Princeton. Darwin-Press. 1978.

A mammoth book designed for scientists, specialists, and laymen with interests in marine biotoxicology and medicine. Book is divided into invertebrates and vertebrates and chapters are by phyla or classes. Glossary of terms. Fully referenced with citations going back to the 19th century. A large chapter of black and white and color plates.

24. Hayes WA. *Mycotoxin Teratogenicity and Mutagenicity.* Boca Raton, FL. CRC Press. 1981.

Among the substances considered are aflatoxins, cytochalasins, ergot alkaloids, fusarium toxins, etc. Combined exposure is also discussed.

25. Kingsbury JM. *Poisonous Plants of the United States and Canada*. Englewood Cliffs, New Jersey. Prentice-Hall. 1964.

A classic text with an extensive bibliography that can be a practical tool for the layman as well as the physician and veterinarian. Photographs and line drawings. Chapters discuss algae, fungi, ferns, horsetails, gymnosperms, and grass tetany. Bacteria are excluded. ''Toxicologically it includes all plants which have caused loss of life and in which toxicity has been traced or may reasonably be traceable to a particular component producing an identifiable or potentially identifiable deleterious reaction in one or more species of animal when taken into the body under natural circumstances.''

26. Lee CY, ed. *Snake Venoms*. Berlin. Springer-Verlag. 1979.

Volume 52 of the *Handbook of Experimental Pharmacology*. Comprehensively reviews research in snake venoms. 28 chapters in 4 parts. Topics covered include history, chemistry, biochemistry, pharmacologic effects, and clinical/immunologic factors.

27. Rodricks JV, Hesseltine CW, Mehlman MA, eds. *Mycotoxins in Human and Animal Health*. Park Forest South, IL. Pathotox. 1977.

Deals with aflatoxins, trichothecenes, and other fusarium toxins, zearalenone, other mycotoxins of possible health significance, biomedical assessment of mycotoxin risks, and regulation and the marketplace. Contains the proceedings of a conference conducted by the United States-Japan Cooperative Program on Natural Resources/Panel on Toxic Microorganisms.

28. Rumack BH, Salzman E, eds. *Mushroom Poisoning: Diagnosis and Treatment*. West Palm Beach, FL. CRC Press. 1978.

Focuses on mushroom identification, mushroom toxicology, and mushroom hallucination. Unique chapter on mushroom worker's lung, a respiratory ailment.

29. Russell FE. *Snake Venom Poisoning*. Philadelphia. Lippincott. 1980.

Of particular interest to physicians, this monograph stresses the biology of venomous snakes, venom poisoning, and treatment. A practical yet scholarly sourcebook augmented with engaging chapters on snakes in mythology, religion, and politics.

30. Uraguchi K, Yamazaki M, eds. *Toxicology, Biochemistry, and Pathology of Mycotoxins*. New York. Halstead. 1978.

The contributors are experts in mycotoxin research. ''The contents are arranged according to the characteristic features and properties of mycotoxins, offering general reviews from the mycological, chemical, toxicological and pathological viewpoints." Specific chapters devoted to carcinogenicity and aflatoxins.

See also:

Keeler RF. *Effects of poisonous plants on livestock.* [under *Veterinary Toxicology*]

Carcinogenesis, Mutagenesis, Teratogenesis

31. Asher IM, Zervos C, eds. *Structural Correlates of Carcinogenesis and Mutagenesis: A Guide to Testing Priorities?* Rockville, MD. US Department of Health, Education, and Welfare, Public Health Service, Food and Drug Administration, Scientific Liason Office, Office of Science. 1977. [HEW Publication Number (FDA)78-1046]

Consists of the proceedings of the second FDA Office of Science Summer Symposium.

32. Berg K, ed. *Genetic Damage in Man Caused by Environmental Agents.* New York. Academic Press. 1979.

Based on a conference arranged by the Norwegian Academy of Science and Letters and others, with an international roster of contributors. Articles arranged in 9 sections: "Inherited Susceptibility," "Point Mutations in Man," "Chromosome Damage," "Sister Chromatid Exchange," "Epidemiologic Approaches," "Biochemical Methods for Monitoring Genetic Damage," "Nonhuman Test Systems," "Antenatal Diagnosis," "Cost of Mutation." An appendix consists of reports of special study groups who have developed reviews of methods for identifying genetic damage.

33. Bowman MC. *Carcinogens and Related Substances: Analytical Chemistry for Toxicological Research.* New York. Marcel Dekker. 1979.

"The purpose of this book is to outline and discuss some of the important principles, problems, and pitfalls encountered in the chemistry of toxicological testing and to provide analytical methodology in sufficient detail to enable a trained chemist to perform many of the assays that may be required."

34. Brusick D. *Principles of Genetic Toxicology.* New York. Plenum Press. 1980.

A welcome new textbook on genetic toxicology focusing on origins and fundamentals of the field, chemical screening for genotoxic properties, genetic risk estimation, environmental/human monitoring, the genetic toxicology lab, and descriptions of assays. The final chapter outlines 21 selected protocols for genetic toxicology. Some of these are the Ames Salmonella Assay, Sister Chromatid Exchange, Chromosome Aberrations, Mouse Micronucleus Assay, Heritable Translocation, etc. Materials, experimental design, procedure, data analysis, and references are among the topics reviewed for each protocol. Appendices on "Preparation of S9 Liver Homogenates", "Dose Selection for in vivo genetic assays" and "Selected References and Reviews of Genetics and Genetic Toxicology."

35. Butterworth BE. *Strategies for Short-Term Testing for Mutagens/ Carcinogens.* Boca Raton, FL. CRC Press. 1979.

Reviews of assays for mutagenicity, DNA damage, etc.

36. Coulston F, Dunne JF, eds. *The Potential Carcinogenicity of Nitrosatable drugs: WHO Symposium, Geneva, June 1978.* Norwood, NJ. Ablex Publishing. 1980.

This is the first volume in the series *Current Topics in Biomedical Research.* Chapters on "Comparative Toxicology of N-Nitroso Compounds and their Carcinogenic Potential to Man," "Potential Health Hazards of Nitrosated Drugs in Perspective," "Pathological Aspects of Nitrosatable Drugs," and others.

37. DeSerres FJ, Fouts JR, Bend JR, Philpot RM, eds. *In Vitro Metabolic Activation in Mutagenesis Testing.* Amsterdam. North-Holland Publishing Company. 1976.

Proceedings of the Symposium on the Role of Metabolic Activation in Producing Mutagenic and Carcinogenic Environmental Chemicals, Research Triangle Park, North Carolina, February 9–11, 1976. Covers indicator organisms, metabolic activation, specific reactions (e.g., activation of benzpyrene, nitrosamines) and DNA interactions.

38. Drake JW, Koch RE, eds. *Mutagenesis.* Stroudsbourg, PA. Hutchinson and Ross. 1976.

Volume 4 in the series *Benchmark Papers in Genetics.* A compilation of classic papers in mutagenesis. The editors provide comments on the papers.

39. Emmelot P, Kriek E. *Environmental Carcinogenesis: Occurrence, Risk Evaluation and Mechanisms.* Amsterdam. Elsevier/North-Holland Biomedical Press. 1979.

Proceedings of the International Conference on Environmental Carcinogenesis held in Amsterdam, May 8–11, 1979. Among the papers in this volume are ones on transplacental carcinogenesis, tumor promotion,

DNA repair, N-nitroso compounds, and interpretation of animal data. The opening paper is by John Higginson of IARC.

40. Epstein S. *Politics of Cancer*. San Francisco. Sierra Book Club Books. 1978.

Views cancer and carcinogenesis from the political, social, economic, legislative, and regulatory perspective. Consumer products, the workplace, the general environment, and governmental policies are some of the more significant topics.

41. Fishbein L. *Potential Industrial Carcinogens and Mutagens*. Amsterdam. Elsevier. 1979.

Volume 4 in the series *Studies in Environmental Science*. Introductory chapters cover combination effects in chemical carcinogenesis, epidemiology, risk assessment and threshold dose, and tabular summaries of potential industrial carcinogens and mutagens. The remaining chapters consider 176 industrial organic chemicals that have been divided into 21 major groups and 38 structural subgroups. Where feasible, mutagenic test systems and carcinogenic responses have been listed.

42. Flamm WG, Mehlman MA, eds. *Mutagenesis*. Washington. Hemisphere. 1978.

Volume 5 of *Advances of Modern Toxicology*. The introductory section discusses mutagenic test systems and guidelines of maximum permissible levels of mutagens. Subsequent sections cover modifying influences (DNA repair, nutrition), test systems for detecting mutations in microorganisms and mammals, sources of natural and synthetic mutagens, and a thorough description of the Environmental Mutagen Information Center.

43. Gelboin HV, Macmahon B, Matsushima T, Sugimura T, Takayama S, Takebe H. *Genetic and Environmental Factors in Experimental and Human Cancer*. Tokyo. Japan Scientific Societies Press. 1980.

Proceedings of the 10th International Symposium of the Princess Takamatsu Cancer Research Fund, Tokyo, 1979. The theme of the symposium was the relationship between genetic and environmental factors in the carcinogenic mechanism. Broad topics include mixed-function oxidases, pharmacogenetics, genetic factors, DNA repair, and epidemiology. Among the papers are those on radiation carcinogenesis in Hiroshima and Nagasaki, cancer among Mormons, and benzo(a)pyrene metabolism.

44. Generoso WM, Shelby MD, de Serres FJ, eds. *DNA Repair and Mutagenesis in Eukaryotes*. New York. Plenum. 1980.

Volume 15 of the series *Basic Life Sciences*. Proceedings of a symposium sponsored by the National Institute of Environmental Health Sciences and held at Atlanta in 1979. Divided into sections on lower eukaryotes, drosophila, mammalian somatic cells, mouse germ cells, and human health hazard assessment.

45. Griffin AC, Shaw CR, eds. *Carcinogens: Identification and Mechanisms of Action*. New York. Raven Press. 1979.

The 31st Annual Symposium on Fundamental Cancer Research of the University of Texas System Cancer Center, M.D. Anderson Hospital and Tumor Institute. Emphasizes detection of environmental carcinogens and the mechanisms by which they induce cancer in the body. Papers on such topics as in vitro chemical carcinogenesis, DNA damage/repair, inhibitors of carcinogenesis, carcinogenesis markers, plasma membrane alterations, and retinoids and cancer prevention.

46. Grover PL, ed. *Chemical Carcinogens and DNA,* 2 volumes. Boca Raton, FL. 1979.

Discusses reaction of DNA with carcinogens, alterations in nucleic acid conformation, and biological effects (e.g., mutagenesis, carcinogenesis) of these reactions and alterations. The editor is with the Institute of Cancer Research, London. The chapters, authored by experts from around the world, provide systematic presentations of important topics and constitute extensive literature reviews.

47. Heinonen OP, Shapiro S, Slone D. *Birth Defects and Drugs in Pregnancy*. Littleton, MA. Publishing Sciences Group. 1977.

"... this book adds substantially to what is known about the general epidemiology of birth defects. It also provides quantitative information . . . concerning relationships between birth defects . . . Perhaps the most important conclusion to emerge with regard to the general epidemiology of malformations is that the etiology of birth defects appears to be multifactorial." Numerous tables and statistical analyses. A unique book relating drugs, teratology, epidemiology, and statistics.

48. Hiatt, HH, Watson JD, Winsten JA, eds. *Origins of Human Cancer*. Cold Spring Harbor, NY. Cold Spring Harbor Laboratory. 1977.

This publication, Volume 4 of the *Cold Spring Harbor Conferences on Cell Proliferation,* has been issued in 3 books: *Incidence of Cancer in Humans, Mechanisms of Carcinogenesis,* and *Human Risk Assessment,* in 19 sections. A large number of papers on short-term assays. Public policy panels on diethylstilbestrol, cyclamates, and dieldrin. A complete and useful conference.

49. Hollaender, A. *Chemical Mutagens: Principles and Methods for Their Detection,* 6 volumes. New York. Plenum Press. 1971–1980.

"The purpose of these volumes is to encourage the development and application of testing and monitoring procedures to avert significant human exposure to mutagenic agents." The volumes are sponsored by the Environmental Mutagen Society.

50. Kilbey BJ, ed. *Handbook of Mutagenicity Test Procedures.* Amsterdam. Elsevier. 1977.

A methodological text designed to provide standard information on conducting a variety of tests to determine genetic damage. Among methods covered are the Ames Salmonella test, yeast systems, micronucleus test, sister chromatid exchange, and drosophila as assay system.

51. Klingberg MA, Weatherall JAC, eds. *Epidemiologic Methods for Detection of Teratogens.* Basel. Karger. 1979.

Volume 1 in the series *Contributions to Epidemiology and Biostatistics.* Presents recent research on environmental teratogens and means for their detection.

52. Kouri RE, ed. *Genetic Differences in Chemical Carcinogenesis.* Boca Raton, FL. CRC Press. 1980.

The authors examine the ways in which genetic variations alter susceptibility to chemically induced cancers. Topics studied include exposure and fate of carcinogens in the body, metabolism of chemical carcinogens, repair of lesions, murine endogenous RNA viruses, two state carcinogenesis, tumor immunology, and host–environmental interaction.

53. Kraybill HF, Mehlman MA, eds. *Environmental Cancer.* Washington, DC. Hemisphere Publishing. 1977.

Volume 3 of *Advances in Modern Toxicology.* Presents an overview of problems related to environmental carcinogenesis. Some of the chapters are "High Pressure Liquid Chromatography: A New Technique for Studying Metabolism and Activation of Chemical Carcinogens," "Conceptual Approaches to the Assessment of Nonoccupational Environmental Cancer," "Occupational Carcinogenesis," "Current Concepts of a Bioassay Program in Environmental Carcinogenesis," "Inorganic Agents as Carcinogens," and "Organohalogen Carcinogens."

54. Mahlum DD, Sikov MR, Hackett PL, Andrew FD, eds. *Developmental Toxicology of Energy-Related Pollutants.* US Department of Energy, Technical Information Center. 1978. [available from NTIS - #CONF-771017].

Consists of proceedings of the 17th Annual Hanford Biology Symposium.

Effects of pollutants generated by new energy technologies on the fetus or immature organism. Papers on gonads, gametes, organic and inorganic pollutants, radiation, human implications, and women workers.

55. Miller EC, Miller JA, Hirono IS, Sugimura T, Takayama S, eds. *Naturally Occurring Carcinogens-Mutagens and Modulators of Carcinogenesis*. Tokyo. Japan Scientic Societies Press. 1979.

Proceedings of the 9th International Symposium of the Princess Takamatsu Cancer Research Fund Tokyo, 1979. An international panel of participants delivered papers on such topics as moldy sweet potatoes, edible plants, brachn fern, defatted soybean, safrole, cooked meats, mushroom, and aflatoxins.

56. Neubert D, Merker H, Kwasigroch TE, eds. *Methods in Prenatal Toxicology*. Stuttgart. Georg Thieme. 1977.

This publication consists of papers presented at a 1977 teratology workshop in Berlin on evaluating embryotoxic effects in experimental animals. Sections on planning experiments, choice of species, evaluation of organ systems and skeletal abnormalities, postnatal manifestation of prenatally induced lesions, in vitro techniques, morphological techniques and biochemical/toxicological techniques in teratology.

57. Nishimura H, Tanimura T. *Clinical Aspects of the Teratogenicity of Drugs*. Amsterdam. Excerpta Medica. 1976.

Discusses concepts of normal and anomalous fetal development, effects of drugs on germ cells and gametogenesis, specific teratogens, prenatal hazards of specific groups of drugs, risks of environmental chemicals to human embryos, etc.

58. Norpoth KH, Garner RC, eds. *Short-Term Test Systems for Detecting Carcinogens*. Berlin. Springer-Verlag. 1980.

Papers on the significance and validity of short-term test systems for carcinogens. In vivo vs in vitro, use of mammalian cells, standardization of procedures, and interpretation of results are topics covered. Papers on combination effects, dog urine testing, antimetabolites, oxygenase-independent activation, biostatistics of Ames Test data, etc.

59. Schmahl D. *Iatrogenic Carcinogenesis*. Berlin. Springer-Verlag. 1977.

Written for pharmacotherapists. An unusual feature is tables of patients by age and sex indicating type of reaction following diagnosis or therapy.

60. Schwartz RH, Yaffe SJ, eds. *Drug and Chemical Risks to the Fetus and Newborn*. New York. Alan R. Liss. 1980.

Volume 36 of *Progress in Clinical and Biological Research*. Topics include "Critical Periods of Prenatal Toxic Insults", "Causal Inference in Teratology," "Male Mediated Effects in Offspring," "The Excretion of Drugs in Milk," and "Neurobehavioral Effects of Prenatal Origin: Sex Hormones."

61. Searle CE, ed. *Chemical Carcinogens*. Washington, DC. American Chemical Society. 1976.

ACS Monograph #173. An extensive survey of chemical carcinogens. Topics include tests and bioassays for chemical carcinogens, endocrine aspects, carcinogens in plants, microorganisms, foods, alkylating agents, soots, tars, oils, N-nitroso compounds. The editors and authors of most of the chapters are English. Extensively referenced.

62. Shaw CR, ed. *Prevention of Occupational Cancer*. Boca Raton, FL. CRC Press. 1981.

Both a scientific overview of carcinogenesis, its mechanism and occupational situation, as well as an analysis of legislation, public education, and regulatory activities.

63. Shepard TH. *Catalog of Teratogenic Agents,* 3rd ed. Baltimore. Johns Hopkins University Press. 1980.

The catalog consists of specific agents and topics related to congenital defects. The author has synthesized the literature into a concise form, provided many summaries, and referenced virtually every statement made.

64. Staffa JA, Mehlman MA, eds. *Innovations in Cancer Risk Assessment (ED01 Study)*. Park Forest South, IL. Pathotox Publishers. 1979.

This low-dose carcinogen study of 2-acetylaminofluorene was conducted with over 24,000 mice. It has important implications for future research in cancer risk assessment.

65. Tuchmann-Duplessis H. *Drug Effects on the Fetus: A Survey of the Mechanisms and Effects of Drugs on Embryogenesis and Fetogenesis*. Sydney. ADIS Press. 1975.

Volume 2 in the series *Monographs on Drugs*. Discusses congenital malformations caused by drugs.

66. Williams GM, Kroes R, Waaijers HW, Van de Poll KW, eds. *The Predictive Value of Short-Term Screening Tests in Carcinogenicity Evaluation*. Amsterdam. Elsevier/North Holland. 1980.

Volume 3 of the series *Applied Methods in Oncology*. This workshop was held in Dalen, the Netherlands in 1980 under the auspices of the Scientific Council of The Netherlands Cancer Society. The scientific basis and validation of various short-term tests for mutagenicity and carcinogenicity were reviewed. International cooperative programs were also described.

67. Wilson JG, Fraser FC. *Handbook of Teratology,* 4 volumes. New York. Plenum Press. 1977.

A comprehensive text covering the following aspects of teratology: Volume 1: "General Principles and Etiology," Volume 2: "Mechanisms and Pathogenesis," Volume 3: "Comparative, Maternal and Epidemiologic Aspects," Volume 4: "Research Procedures and Data Analysis."

See also:

Coulston F, ed. *Regulatory Aspects of Carcinogenesis and Food Additives: the Delaney Clause.* [under *Legislative, Regulatory, and Societal Issues*]

Gelboin HV. *Polycyclic Hydrocarbons and Cancer.* [under *Environmental Toxicology*]

Hart RW, ed. *A Rational Evaluation of Pesticidal vs. Mutagenic/Carcinogenic Action.* [under *Pesticides*]

Hayes, WA. *Mycotoxin Teratogenicity and Mutagenicity.* [under *Biotoxins*]

Kraybill HF, ed. *Aquatic Pollutants and Biologic Effects with Emphasis on Neoplasia.* [under *Environmental Toxicology*]

Lapis K. *Liver Carcinogenesis.* [under *Target Systems*]

Schardein JL. *Drugs as Teratogens.* [under *Drugs*]

Schwarz RH, ed. *Drug and Chemical Risks to the Fetus and Newborn.* [under *Drugs*]

Sigel H, ed. *Carcinogenicity and Metal Ions.* [under *Metals*]

Chapter on Special Monographs

Clinical Toxicology

68. American Academy of Pediatrics. *Handbook of Common Poisonings in Children.* Rockville, MD. US Department of Health, Education and Welfare, Public Health Service, Food and Drug Administration. 1976.

Brief volume limiting itself to the 73 toxic substances most often responsible for accidental poisoning of children. A practical guide.

69. Ansell G. *Radiology in Clinical Toxicology.* London. Butterworth. 1974.

Diagnostic radiology used in the detection of hazardous substances in the body is the topic. Serves as a reference for clinicians and a handbook for radiologists.

70. Arena JM. *Poisoning: Toxicology-Symptoms-Treatments*, 4th ed. Spring-field, IL. Charles C. Thomas. 1979.

> Compilation of valuable information. General considerations of poison-ing, pesticides, industrial and occupational hazards, drugs, cosmetics, and poisonous plants and animals are all covered. A practical book on product descriptions, diagnosis, and treatments. In addition to coverage of most of the frequently involved chemical poisons, such unlikely topics as crayons, golf balls, and toxic Christmas decorations are discussed. An appendix with sources of popular posters, booklets, and audiovisuals. Directory of US poison control centers.

71. Baselt RC. *Disposition of Toxic Drugs and Chemicals in Man*. Canton, CT. Biomedical Publications. 1978.

> Presents "information on the disposition of the chemicals and drugs most frequently encountered in episodes of human poisoning. The data in-cluded relate to the body fluid concentrations of substances in normal and therapeutic situations, concentrations in fluids and tissues in instances of toxicity and the known metabolic fate of these substances in man."

72. Brown VK. *Acute Toxicity in Theory and Practice: With Special Reference to the Toxicology of Pesticides*. Chichester. John Wiley. 1980.

> "This book is orientated towards the general principles of acute toxicol-ogy while utilizing the fact that the diverse properties of pesticides pro-vide a plethora of examples to illustrate these principles.

73. Curry AS. *Advances in Forensic and Clinical Toxicology*. Cleveland. Chemical Rubber Company. 1972.

> Discusses analysis of chemicals and classes of chemicals generally known to be abused or hazardous.

74. Curry AS. *Poison Detection in Human Organs,* 3rd ed. Springfield, IL. Charles C. Thomas. 1976.

> Forensic toxicology. This book "assumes that the analyst is pitting his wits against the criminal poisoner and that the capsules or medicine left by the side of the bed are not the ones taken in the accidental or suicidal overdose case." Both the living and the dead are subjects for analysis.

75. Czajka PA, Duffy JP. *Poisoning Emergencies: A Guide for Emergency Medical Personnel*. St. Louis, MO. CV Mosby. 1980.

> A pocket guide to poisoning by various substances. Information provided includes common products in which the substance is an ingredient, routes of exposure, symptoms, potential complications, prehospital and hospital treatment, and references. Table on plant poisonings. Glossary of drug

abuse terms (e.g., "Monroe in a Cadillac" = a mixture of morphine and cocaine).

76. De Castro FJ, Jaeger W. *Clinical Toxicology Manual*. St. Louis, MO. Catholic Hospital Association. 1978.

A concise manual for the practitioner in emergency rooms and hospital wards.

77. Dreisbach RH. *Handbook of Poisoning: Diagnosis and Treatment*. 10th ed. Los Altos, CA. Lange. 1980.

"A concise summary of the diagnosis and treatment of clinically important poisons." General considerations, agricultural poisons, industrial hazards, household hazards, medicinal poisons, animal and plant hazards. Over 800 recent references in this compact handbook.

78. Goldfrank LR, Kirstein R. *Toxicologic Emergencies: A Handbook in Problem Solving*. New York. Appleton-Century-Crofts. 1978.

Emphasis on diagnosis, not therapy, in the emergency room. Problem oriented with numerous case studies.

79. Gosselin RE, Hodge HC, Smith RP, Gleason MN. *Clinical Toxicology of Commercial Products*. 4th ed. Baltimore. Williams and Wilkins. 1976.

A standard reference work in clinical toxicology, "the purpose of this book is to assist the physician in dealing quickly and effectively with acute chemical poisonings, arising through misuse of commercial products." The seven sections of the book, color coded for easy access, are: 1. First Aid and General Emergency Treatment; 2. Ingredients Index (including toxicity ratings for chemical substances); 3. Therapeutics Index (concentrates on toxic signs and symptoms plus therapy for compounds and classes of compounds); 4. Supportive Treatment; 5. Trade Name Index (this is a product composition and manufacturer identification file); 6. General Formulations (a guide to the probable composition of products not specifically listed by brand name in section 5; 7. Manufacturers Index (a handy listing with phone numbers when available). Kept up to date by monthly "Bulletin of Supplementary Material". This publication is computer searchable on the NIH-EPA system.

80. Hanenson IB, ed. *Quick Reference to Clinical Toxicology*. Philadelphia. JB Lippincott. 1980.

Designed as a ready reference tool for the physician who must identify and manage toxic drug effects. 23 contributors have provided chapters on various classes of compounds, interactions, toxicologic information, and analytic methods.

81. Kaye S. *Handbook of Emergency Toxicology*. 4th ed. Springfield, IL. Charles C. Thomas. 1980.

A fine handbook on ''the problems involved in the rapid presumptive diagnosis and treatment of 'alleged' poisoning.'' The main portion of the book alphabetically lists poisons, their synonyms, uses, MLDs symptoms of acute and chronic toxicity, identification, and treatment. Another large chapter is on analysis and describes techniques such as acid-steam distillation, microdiffusion, UV, chromatography, etc. Additionally, there are chapters on antidotes/treatment and symptoms/signs, the latter of which lists potential poisons and diseases that may be the causes of various symptoms.

82. Lowry WT, Garriott JC. *Forensic Toxicology: Controlled Substances and Dangerous Drugs*. New York. Plenum Press, 1979.

The major section of this monograph is a listing of substances listed in the Controlled Substances Act, along with certain other dangerous drugs. Synonyms, pharmaceutical preparations, general comments, biochemistry, and toxicology-pharmacology are included with most entries. Additional chapters on dosage forms, regulation of controlled substances, excluded and excepted substances, drug isomers, and instrumentation for analysis of drugs.

83. *Medical First Aid Guide for Use in Accidents Involving Dangerous Goods*. London. Inter-Governmental Maritime Consultative Organization. 1973.

Contains ''recommendations for medical first aid to be given after accidents and for preventive measures against poisoning connected with the carriage of dangerous goods.''

84. Oliver JS, ed. *Forensic Toxicology*. London. Croom Helm. 1980.

Proceedings of the European Meeting of the International Association of Forensic Toxicologists. A wide-ranging group of papers in subjects such as insulin murders, extractive dialysis, plasma paraquat assays, analysis of blood in glue sniffing cases, analysis of blood volatiles from fire fatalaties, pesticide screening, mercury intoxication, and the detection of drugs in greyhound urine.

85. *Sourcebook for Regional and Satellite Poison Centers*. Pittsburgh. National Poison Center Network. 1977.

A brief and lucid examination of the problems facing poison control centers today plus suggested solutions. Discussion of treatment, regionalization, education, communications, and funding.

86. Tedeschi CG, Eckert WG, Tedeschi LG, eds. *Forensic Medicine: A Study* *in Trauma and Environmental Hazards. Volume 3: Environmental Hazards.* Philadelphia. WB Saunders. 1977.

Volumes 1 and 2 of this text are on mechanical and physical trauma, respectively. Volume 3 will be of particular interest to both the legal and medical professions. Presents scientific data, case studies, and information on medical litigation. Several chapters are devoted to legal theories relevant to hazards. These are negligence, malpractice, product liability, causation, damages, informed consent, and workmen's claims.

87. Thienes CH, Haley TJ. *Clinical Toxicology,* 5th ed. Philadelphia. Lea and Febiger. 1972.

Intended as a textbook, this work groups poisons according to major toxic action (e.g., convulsant poisons, central nervous system depressants, etc.). There is generally no detailed discussion of the chemistry or pharmacology of the poisons. Symptoms, diagnosis, and treatment is stressed.

88. Wilber CG. *Forensic Toxicology for the Law Enforcement Officer.* Springfield, IL. Charles C. Thomas. 1980.

Provides a generalized account of toxicology for law enforcement officers, by describing topics such as suicide, abused drugs, alcohol, riot control chemicals, and toxic gases. Tables on alcoholic disorders and alcohol consumption, blood level data of chemicals, and minimum lethal dose of certain volatile hydrocarbons.

89. Woolley BH, Temple AR, eds. *Toxicology and Poison Prevention.* Miami. Symposia Specialists Medical Books. 1977.

''The first section provides an overview of the general principles in toxicology. The second section is a compendium of management of specific types of poisoning.''

See also:

D'Arcy PF. *Drug-Induced Emergencies.* [under *Drugs*]

Gottschalk LA. *Toxicological and Pathological Studies on Drug-Involved Deaths.* [under *Drugs*]

Needleman HL. *Low Level Lead Exposure.* [under *Metals*]

Nishimura H. *Clinical Aspects of the Teratogenicity of Drugs.* [under *Carcinogenesis, Mutagenesis, Teratogenesis*]

Cosmetics

90. Estrin NF, ed. *CTFA Cosmetic Ingredient Dictionary.* Washington, DC. Cosmetic, Toiletry and Fragrance Association, 1980.

Provides nomenclature for ingredients used by cosmetic manufacturers. Chemical structures are displayed. Substance name and supplier indexes.

91. Opdyke DLJ. *Monographs on Fragrance Raw Materials*. In *Food and Cosmetics Toxicology* 17(Suppl 5), Dec 1979. Oxford. Pergamon Press.

Compilation of data on individual fragrance components. Unfavorable and favorable results are presented in the monographs. Excellent source for the toxicities of these products. Referenced.

92. US Congress. House Committee on Interstate and Foreign Commerce. Subcommittee on Oversight and Investigations. *Safety of Hair Dyes and Cosmetic Products*. Hearings, 96th Congress, First Session. Washington, DC. US Government Printing Office. 1979. [Serial #96-105]

Includes testimony of individuals from such groups as the American Academy of Dermatology, AFL-CIO, National Cancer Institute, and the Environmental Defense Fund. Statement submitted by the Cosmetic, Toiletry, and Fragrance Association, Inc. Also contains a doctoral dissertation on "Cancer Incidence Amongst Cosmetologists." According to the subcommittee chairman "the subcommittee found that American men and women put an average of 10 to 40 pounds of powder, perfumes, toiletries, and soaps on their skins annually and that as much as several pounds of the chemicals in these cosmetics can penetrate the skin and be absorbed into the bloodstream."

See also:

Drill VA. *Cutaneous Toxicity*. [under *Target Systems*]

Grant WM. *Toxicology of the Eye*. [under *Target Systems*]

Leung AY. *Encyclopedia of Common Natural Ingredients*. [under *Food*]

Marzulli F. *Dermatotoxicology and Pharmacology*. [under *Target Systems*]

Mokler BV. *Inhalation Toxicology Studies of Aerosolized Products*. [under *Environmental Toxicology*]

Simon GA. *Skin: Drug Application and Evaluation of Environmental Hazards*. [under *Target Systems*]

Smith MB. *Handbook of Ocular Toxicity*. [under *Target Systems*]

Drugs

93. AMA Department of Drugs. *AMA Drug Evaluations*, 4th ed. New York. American Medical Association. 1980.

Information is provided on drugs used clinically. Includes data on structure, description, dosage forms, routes, adverse reactions, interactions.

Three chapters devoted to "Drug Antidotes in Poisoning." Prepared by the AMA's Department of Drugs in cooperation with the American Society for Clinical Pharmacology and Therapeutics.

94. D'Arcy PF, Griffin JP, eds. *Drug-induced Emergencies.* Bristol. John Wright. 1980.

The authors warn that "the prescriber should always be aware that the combination of a drug and a patient is a potential emergency looking for someone to happen to." Among the topics covered are emergencies in anaesthetic practice, allergic emergencies, emergencies presenting as acute surgical problems, drug-induced neurological and psychiatric syndromes, drug-induced cytopenias, disorders of coagulation, infection, and cardiovascular emergencies. Chapter on oculo- and oto-toxicity plus an index of official and proprietary names.

95. D'Arcy PF, Griffin JP, eds. *Iatrogenic Diseases,* 2nd ed. Oxford. Oxford University Press. 1979.

Drug-induced diseases throughout the body are discussed. Includes acute and chronic effects, metabolic disturbances, endocrine dysfunction, etc. Chapter on hazards of vaccines. Appendices on drug interactions and cross-index of names—proprietary and official.

96. Davies DM, ed. *Textbook of Adverse Drug Reactions.* Oxford. Oxford University Press. 1977.

Edited by the editor of the *Adverse Drug Reaction Bulletin.* Most of the contributors are affiliated with the Newcastle Medical School. Basically organized by site of disorder, e.g., chromosome, cardiac, respiratory, dental, gastrointestinal, hepatic, renal, metabolic, skin, etc. Includes chapters on drug allergies, topical antiseptics, opaque media, and medico-legal aspects.

97. Dukes MNG, ed. *Meyler's Side Effects of Drugs: An Encyclopaedia of Adverse Reactions and Interactions,* 9th ed. Amsterdam. Excerpta Medica. 1980.

The new edition of this classic reference tool has been entirely revamped and rewritten with all older references checked for reliability. Many have been dropped and new more relevant ones added. Drugs are classified in 51 different families. For each family or specific drug representative of a family, a consistently organized monograph is offered. The data in each of these monographs contains information on such topics as adverse reaction patterns, effects on organs and systems, risk situations, withdrawal effects, effects on genes and the fetus, overdosage, interactions, and interference with diagnostic routines. Includes a list of synonyms and an international compilation of "National centres for adverse reaction monitoring.'' Overall, an elegant, precisely edited publication of exceptional practical value. A companion to this is the serial *Side Effects of Drugs Annual.*

98. Gilman AG, Goodman LS, Gilman A, eds. *Goodman and Gilman's The Pharmacological Basis of Therapeutics,* 6th ed. New York. Macmillan. 1980.

A standard in pharmacology, this text offers extensive coverage of pharmacology, toxicology, and therapeutics. Most of the chapters of this new edition have been either totally rewritten or revised. Following general principles of therapeutics and pharmacodynamics, chapters concentrate on drugs acting on various bodily systems, organs and diseases. Hormones and vitamins are included. A new section of 3 chapters is devoted to toxicology. In addition to chemistry, pharmacological actions, dosages, absorption and fate, specific entries for drugs offer such information as toxicity (acute and chronic), side effects, hypersensitivity, etc., where applicable. Appendixes on prescription order writing, dosage regimens, and drug interactions.

99. Goldstein A, Aronow L, Kalman SM. *Principles of Drug Action: the Basis of Pharmacology,* 2nd ed. New York. John Wiley and Sons. 1974.

This book on drug action places toxicology firmly within the scope of pharmacology. After basic principles of absorption, distribution, metabolism, and excretion are covered, the authors devote a substantial portion of the text to drug toxicity, mutagenesis, teratogenesis, carcinogenesis, allergy, resistance, and tolerance.

100. Gorrod JW, ed. *Drug Toxicity.* London. Taylor and Francis. 1979.

Devotes chapters to toxic products, developmental features of drug toxicity, effects of genetics, diet, and differences in formulation in drug toxicity, and enzyme induction. Also discussed is neurotoxic responses, cancer induction, teratogenesis, skin reactions, eye reactions, and effects of drugs on the pulmonary system.

101. Gottschalk LA, Cravey RH. *Toxicological and Pathological Studies on Psychoactive Drug-involved Deaths.* Davis, CA. Biomedical Publications. 1980.

A research team from UCLA collected data from the medical examiners and coroners of nine major cities, on psychoactive drug involved deaths. For each drug, the data tabulated in this book includes the route of administration, the role of the drug in death, ICDA codes, a physical description of the deceased, autopsy findings, and toxicological findings. Information provided for toxicological findings are the site assayed, the concentration of drug found, methods of extraction and analysis, and extraction pH. Introductory chapters cover the statistical data collection procedures, details of the toxicological examinations, and the uses of toxicological data.

102. Martin EW. *Hazards of Medication,* 2nd ed. Philadelphia. JB Lippincott Company. 1978.

A comprehensive volume devoted to hazards in prescribing and taking medications. The Table of Drug Interactions is a thoroughly documented listing of ''drug interactions published since 1955 in the world medical literature for more than 1000 of the most widely prescribed drugs, including the 200 drugs most frequently prescribed in the United States.'' Chapters on research and development, manufacturing, distribution and storage, and prescribing factors.

103. Preger L, ed. *Induced Disease: Drug, Irradiation, Occupation.* New York. Grune and Stratton. 1980.

Short papers on a wide range of induced diseases. Of particular interest to practicing clinicians and radiologists. The contributors are primarily radiologists and the book, overall, even the chapters on drug and occupational diseases, has a strong radiographic emphasis. Numerous radiographs, conventional and CAT scans, are provided to illustrate pathology.

104. Roe DA. *Drug-Induced Nutritional Deficiencies.* Westport, CT. AVI Publishing Company. 1976.

Examines mechanisms by which drugs induce nutritional disorders. Topics such as drug-induced malnutrition and malabsorption, antivitamins and fetal malnutrition are discussed in addition to specific effects of alcohol, anticonvulsants, oral contraceptives, antituberculosis drugs, and anti-Parkinson drugs.

105. Schardein JL. *Drugs as Teratogens.* Cleveland. CRC Press. 1976.

''Part I deals with the problem of drug consumption by the pregnant woman and with laboratory assessment of this hazard. Part II is concerned with the teratogenic properties of drugs in animals and in man.'' Over 1200 therapeutic agents are discussed with relevant references through 1975 included. Photographs of birth defects. Discussion of drugs divided into chapters by their action.

106. Schwarz RH, Yaffe SJ, eds. *Drug and Chemical Risks to the Fetus and Newborn.* New York. Alan R. Liss. 1980.

Proceedings of a symposium held in New York City, May 1979, sponsored by the National Foundation–March of Dimes. Papers on both acute and long term effects of agents administered either prenatally or via breast milk exposure.

107. Soda T, ed. *Drug-Induced Sufferings: Medical, Pharmaceutical and Legal Aspects.* Amsterdam. Excerpta Medica. 1980.

Proceedings of the Kyoto International Conference Against Drug-Induced Sufferings, April 14–18, 1979, Kyoto, Japan. Papers presented via keynote reports, 3 sessions (covering medical and pharmaceutical aspects, and legal and social aspects), a panel discussion on SMON (subacute myelo-optico-neuropathy) and a plenary session. Provides interesting perspectives from a number of countries.

108. Wade A, ed. *Martindale: The Extra Pharmacopoeia,* 27th ed. London. The Pharmaceutical Press. 1977.

Lengthy monographs on drugs and related substances. Includes toxic effects. References are abstracted. A good source for the identification of drugs. Section on proprietary medicines. Includes a directory of manufacturers, an index to clinical uses, and a detailed subject index.

109. Windholz M, ed. *The Merck Index: An Encyclopedia of Chemicals and Drugs,* 9th ed. Rahway, NJ. Merck and Company. 1976.

Monographs on some 10,000 substances known by more than 50,000 synonyms. Chemical structures are often provided. Patent information. Literature references. Miscellaneous appendices on organic name reactions, first aid in poison incidents, manufacturer directory, tables of weights and measures, list of Chemical Abstracts registry numbers. Formula and name indexes.

110. Zbinden G, Gross F. *Pharmacological Methods in Toxicology.* Oxford. Pergamon. 1979.

This is section 102 of the *International Encyclopedia of Pharmacology and Therapeutics* and was published as a supplement to the journal *Pharmacology and Therapeutics.* Deals "mainly with disturbances of organ function, which often are undesired companions of the beneficial actions of drugs." 10 chapters cover topics that include cadiovascular, autonomic, gastrointestinal, behavioral, and neuropsycho-, pharmacologies.

See also:

Albert A. *Selective Toxicity.* [under *Miscellaneous*]

Baselt RC. *Disposition of Toxic Drugs and Chemicals in Man.* [under *Clinical Toxicology*]

Coulston F. *The Potential Carcinogenicity of Nitrosatable Drugs.* [under *Carcinogenesis, Mutagenesis, Teratogenesis*]

Davidson CS. *Guidelines for Detection of Hepatotoxicity due to Drugs and Chemicals.* [under *Target Systems*]

Heinonen OP. *Birth Defects and Drugs in Pregnancy.* [under *Carcinogenesis, Mutagenesis, Teratogenesis*]

Nishimura H. *Clinical Aspects of the Teratogenicity of Drugs.* [under *Carcinogenesis, Mutagenesis, Teratogenesis*]

Schmahl D. *Iatrogenic Carcinogenesis.* [under *Carcinogenesis, Mutagenesis, Teratogenesis*]

Schwartz RH. *Drug and Chemical Risks to the Fetus and Newborn.* (under *Carcinogenesis, Mutagenesis, Teratogenesis*)

Tuchmann-Duplessis H. *Drug Effects on the Fetus.* [under *Carcinogenesis, Mutagenesis, Teratogenesis*]

Section on *Analytical Toxicology*

Environmental Toxicology

111. Berlin A, Wolff AH, Hasegawa Y. *The Use of Biological Specimens for the Assessment of Human Exposure to Environmental Pollutants.* The Hague. Nijhoff. 1979.

> Proceedings of a symposium held at Luxembourg in 1977 and jointly organized by the Commission of the European Communities, EPA, and WHO. Among the objectives were "to assess the types of environmental pollutants and human specimens most suitable for 'biological monitoring' and to evaluate the probable usefulness of biological specimen banking" and "to examine the state of the art and the technical feasibility of programmes designed to collect, analyze and store samples relative to biological monitoring and biological specimen banking." The general workshop report is followed by the working papers. Includes table showing major environmental pollutants and human tissues, organs and fluids that could be collected for biological monitoring.

112. Bhatnagar RS, ed. *Molecular Basis of Environmental Toxicity.* Ann Arbor, MI. Ann Arbor Science. 1980.

> Papers discuss the interaction of living cells with environmental agents. Sections on "Free Radical Mechanisms," "Mechanisms of Cellular Injury," "Molecular Mechanisms in Environmental Carcinogenesis," "Metal-Tissue Interaction," "Environmental Effects on Macromolecular Structure," and "Problems in Correlating Molecular Mechanisms with Environmental Toxicity."

113. Calabrese EJ. *Pollutants and High-Risk Groups.* New York. John Wiley. 1978.

> Part of the *Environmental Science and Technology* series of monographs. Concentrates on effects of pollutants on especially susceptible portions of the population. High risk groups are identified with an eye to facilitate standard setting and environmental health policy. Groups that

are at high risk as a result of developmental processes, genetic disorders, nutritional deficiencies, etc., are discussed. Informative tables including one for each listed high-risk group identifying the population affected and the pollutant to which the group may be susceptible. Glossary. Bibliography. Subject and author indexes.

114. Cattabeni F, Cavallaro A, Galli G, eds. *Dioxin: Toxicological and Chemical Aspects*. New York. Spectrum Publications. 1978.

Volume 1 in the *Monographs of the Giovanni Lorenzini Foundation*. Opens with a review of the Seveso accident in which a mixture of chemicals containing dioxin was released. Subsequent papers are on the chemistry, toxicology, and decontamination of dioxin.

115. De Bruin A. *Biochemical Toxicology of Environmental Agents*. Amsterdam. Elsevier. 1976.

A comprehensive treatment of "biochemistry applied to occupational and environmental toxicology." 42 chapters, 13,000 references, and a subject index. Radiation effects are discussed at the end of each chapter. Emphasis on metabolism.

116. Duffus JH. *Environmental Toxicology*. London. Edward Arnold. 1980.

In this brief introduction to the subject, "the author uses an interdisciplinary approach to the analysis of environmental effects of toxic substances by first dealing with the assessment of toxicity, then describing the metabolism of toxicants by animals, plants, and micro-organisms and discussing the present knowledge of toxicants of current concern."

117. Fouts JR, Gut I, eds. *Industrial and Environmental Xenobiotics: In vitro versus in vivo Biotransformation and Toxicity*. Amsterdam. Excerpta Medica. 1978.

Number 440 in the *International Congress Series,* this represents the proceedings of an international conference held in Prague in 1977. "The purpose of this conference was therefore to improve understanding of the applicability of in vitro biotransformation data to the living organism, the relationship between hepatic and extrahepatic biotransformation rates, disposition and excretion of xenobiotics, and the applicability of drug biotransformation data to the biotransformation and toxicological studies of industrial and environmental xenobiotics."

117a. Gelboin HV, Ts'o POP, eds. *Polycyclic Hydrocarbons and Cancer*. New York. Academic Press, 1978.

In 2 volumes, summarizes work done in polycyclic aromatic hydrocarbons and cancer. Some of the topics covered are energy sources, environmental occurrence, tobacco carcinogenesis, enzymology, pharmacokinetics, microbial and mammalian mutagenesis, DNA repair, animal and human models, and genetics.

118. Hammond EC, Selikoff IJ, eds. *Public Control of Environmental Hazards.* New York. New York Academy of Sciences. 1979.

Volume 329 of *Annals of the New York Academy of Sciences,* based on a conference held at the Academy in June 1978. An enlightening treatment of environmental health hazards from both the scientific and public policy viewpoints. Includes papers on individual freedom and social control, risk-benefit analyses, constraints in the rationalization of social response to environmental hazards. Included is a series of articles by media reporters on news coverage of environmental hazards. Conference panel discussions and debates have been transcribed as well.

119. Haque R, ed. *Dynamics, Exposure and Hazard Assessment of Toxic Chemicals.* Ann Arbor, MI. Ann Arbor Science. 1980.

Concentrates on transport and fate of toxic chemicals in the environment. Several papers relating to TSCA and transport/fate studies. Other papers present mathematical/computer/system models for describing the behavior of chemicals in the ecosystem. Toxicological dynamics, aquatic hazard evaluation, vapor behavior of toxic organics, and organic photochemistry are among the many other topics considered.

120. *Health Hazards of the Human Environment.* Geneva. World Health Organization. 1972.

WHO's examination of environmental health hazards looks at ''The Community Environment,'' ''Chemical Contaminants and Physical Hazards,'' ''Surveillance and Monitoring,'' and ''Public Health Principles and Practices of Intervention.'' Contributors to and reviewers of this document include specialists from around the world.

121. *Human Health and the Environment: Some Research Needs. Report of the Second Task Force for Research and Planning in Environmental Health Science.* Washington, DC. US Department of Health, Education, and Welfare, Public Health Service, National Institutes of Health, National Institute of Environmental Health Sciences. 1977. [DHEW Publication #NIH 77-1277]

The task force has examined all aspects of environmental health research from atmospheric pollution to transport to carcinogenesis to behavioral toxicology to risk to professional education. Each chapter offers a review of research, specific recommendations, and lists of background documents, references, and other relevant material.

122. Kates RW. *Risk Assessment of Environmental Hazard.* Chichester. John Wiley. 1978.

Published on behalf of the Scientific Committee on Problems of the Environment (SCOPE) of the International Council of Scientific Unions (ICSU). An interesting, systematic, rational, and literate approach to hazards and risk assessment. Case studies from Canada, Africa, Sweden, the USSR, and the US are discussed. Good list of references.

123. Khan MAQ, Bederka JP Jr, eds. *Survival in Toxic Environments.* New York. Academic Press. 1974.

Based on a symposium organized by the American Society of Zoologists. Discusses hazardous environmental chemicals. Topics include pesticides, petroleum, PCBs, polycyclic aromatic hydrocarbons, lead, and carbon monoxide. "The dispositions of these substances and the effects of certain of them were studied in either ecosystems and/or organisms, or components thereof."

124. Koeman JH, Strik JJTWA, eds. *Sublethal Effects of Toxic Chemicals on Aquatic Animals.* Amsterdam. Elsevier. 1975.

Proceedings of the Swedish-Netherlands Symposium, Wageningen, The Netherlands. September 2–5, 1975. Some of the chemicals discussed in their uptake by aquatic organisms are cadmium, mercury, chromium, lead, zinc, PCBs, hexachlorobutadiene, chloronaphthalenes, and dieldren.

125. Kraybill HF, Dawe CJ. Harshbarger JC, Tardiff RG, eds. *Aquatic Pollutants and Biological Effects with Emphasis on Neoplasia.* New York. New York Academy of Sciences. 1977.

Volume 298 of the *Annals of the New York Academy of Sciences.* As the title suggests, the stress in this monograph, consisting of papers of a conference, is on neoplasms in aquatic animals. Mollusks, eels, salamanders, carp, hagfish, and trout are among the animals on which papers were presented. Other topics discussed were implications for man of biological effects on marine animals, and public health aspects.

126. Laskin S, Goldstein BD. *A Critical Evaluation of Benzene Toxicity.* New York. New York University Medical Center, Institute of Environmental Medicine. 1977.

Prepared under contract for the American Petroleum Institute. Reviews analysis, metabolism, experimental intoxication, cytologic effects, and hematotoxicity. Extensive list of references.

127. Lee DHK, ed. *Reactions to Environmental Agents.* Bethesda, MD. American Physiological Society. 1977.

Section 9 of the *Handbook of Physiology*. Divided into the following parts: "Response to Physical Agents", "Nature, Origin, and Distribution of Chemical Agents", "Reactions and Determinants at Portal of Entry", "Transportation and Transformation of Chemical Agents", "Distribution and Excretion of Chemical Agents and Derivatives", and "Mechanism of Cellular Injury".

128. Lee SD, ed. *Biochemical Effects of Environmental Pollutants*. Ann Arbor, MI. Ann Arbor Science. 1977.

Papers examining the biochemical mechanisms by which chemical pollutants produce disease. Most of the studies discuss either trace metal or oxidant pollutant toxicology.

129. Lee SD, ed. *Nitrogen Oxides and Their Effects on Health*. Ann Arbor, MI. Ann Arbor Science. 1980.

After several papers on nitrogen oxide monitoring, the remainder of the book contains reviews on effects of the chemical on experimental animals and on humans. Among the many papers of interest are those on indoor NO_2 exposure, effects of low-level exposures on pulmonary function, and combination effects with ozone in mice.

130. Lefaux R. *Practical Toxicology of Plastics*. London. Iliffe Books. 1968.

Covers chemistry, toxicology, industrial hygiene, surgical applications, and food toxicology of plastics and high polymers. Includes legislative appendices for 5 countries.

131. Lippmann M, Schlesinger RB. *Chemical Contamination and the Human Environment*. New York. Oxford University Press. 1979.

A thorough and valuable overview of how chemicals effect the total environment. It "has been prepared as a text for an introductory graduate level course given in the Interdepartmental Program in Environmental Health Sciences of the Graduate School of Arts and Science of New York University." Dispersion, fate, and sources of contaminants are discussed as well as sampling and measurement and health effects.

132. Mayer FL, Hamelink JL, eds. *Aquatic Toxicology and Hazard Evaluation*. Philadelphia. American Society for Testing and Materials. 1977.

Proceedings of the First Annual Symposium on Aquatic Toxicology. The Symposium covered areas such as toxicity testing, residue dynamics, and biological effects.

133. Mokler BV, Damon EG, Henderson TR, Carpenter RL, Benjamin SA, Rebar AH, Jones RK. *Inhalation Toxicology Studies of Aerosolized Products: Final Report*. Albuquerque, NM. Lovelace Biomedical and En-

vironmental Research Institute, Inhalation Toxicology Research Institute.
1979. [Available from NTIS - #PB80-108509]

> Based on research supported by the FDA and CPSC, on aerosolized
> cosmetics and household products. Research includes "experimental
> studies of the physical and chemical nature of aerosols generated during
> the use of aerosolized products, the deposition and retention charac-
> teristics of representative product ingredients when inhaled by small
> animals, and the biological effects of these materials after repeated inha-
> lation exposure. A general approach has been developed to unify the
> experimental observations and apply them to the assessment of the
> human health risk arising from the use of aerosolized products."

134. National Research Council. *Decisionmaking for Regulating Chemicals in
the Environment*. Washington, DC. National Academy of Sciences. 1975.

> An analysis of the federal regulatory decisionmaking process as it
> applies to industrial chemicals. Discussion of cost-benefit analysis. Ap-
> pendices consist of working papers of a committee on decision making
> and cover topics such as information needs, regulatory options, equity,
> the public. Serves as a companion volume to the Academy's *Principles
> for Evaluating Chemicals in the Environment*.

135. National Research Council. *Principles for Evaluating Chemicals in the
Environment*. Washington, DC. National Academy of Sciences. 1975.

> A key-document that addresses basic issues of safety assessment. Some
> topics discussed are testing, risk-benefit analysis, estimation of exposure
> levels, human health effects, acute, subchronic, chronic toxicities plus
> carcinogenesis, mutagenesis, teratogenesis, and behavioral effects.
> Chapters also devoted to nonhuman biological effects, inanimate sys-
> tems, analysis, and monitoring. Seven appendices and supplementary
> material to the chapters. Extensive references and suggested readings.
> This is not a mere listing of toxic agents but a thoughtful analysis of
> some critical issues in toxicology.

136. National Research Council. *Principles and Procedures for Evaluating the
Toxicity of Household Substances*. Washington, DC. National Academy of
Sciences. 1977.

> For use by the professional toxicologist as administrator or scientific
> investigator. Approaches to testing household products for various
> toxicities—ingestion, skin and eye, inhalation, carcinogenesis,
> mutagenesis, teratogenesis, and behavioral—are discussed. Test prepa-
> rations, procedures, and evaluations are described for animals and hu-
> mans.

137. National Research Council. Safe Drinking Water Committee. *Drinking*

Water and Health. Washington, DC. National Academy of Sciences. 1977.

A thorough "assessment of the long-term biological effects of ingesting the variety of different materials that are present in trace amounts in drinking water." After a general discussion of safety and risk factors in chemical contaminants, chapters are devoted to microbiology, solid particles, inorganic solutes, and radioactivity, all as they are related to drinking water. Numerous references. The most complete treatment on this subject.

138. Nicholson WJ, Moore JA, eds. *Health Effects of Halogenated Aromatic Hydrocarbons.* New York. New York Academy of Sciences. 1979.

Consists of papers in areas such as animal and human health effects, neurologic toxicities, carcinogenesis, reproductive hazards, immunologic abnormalities, and surveillance. Several papers consider the problem of PCBs in the Hudson River as a case study.

139. Peters GA, Peters BJ. *Sourcebook on Asbestos Diseases: Medical, Legal, and Engineering Aspects.* New York. Garland STPM Press. 1980.

A thorough reference guide to asbestos and asbestos-related diseases. Includes list of trade associations, manufacturers of control equipment, annotated legal cases, standards for various countries, an annotated chronological bibliography, and a 1979 postscript outlining recent important issues.

140. Preger L. *Asbestos-Related Disease.* New York. Grune and Stratton. 1978.

"One of the major attractions of the book is the close attention paid to a correlation of the epidemiologic, pathogenetic, pathological, roentgenologic, and clinical manifestations of asbestos related disease." Clinical and microscopic features of various organs involved in asbestos-related disease are described.

141. Selikoff IJ, Hammond EC, eds. *Health Hazards of Asbestos Exposure.* New York. New York Academy of Sciences. 1979.

Volume 330 of the *Annals of the New York Academy of Sciences.* Both occupational and other environmental exposures are covered. Discussions on epidemiology, regulations, standard setting, the shipyard industry, mesothelioma, high-risk groups, and interactions.

142. Smith RL, Bababunmi EA, eds. *Toxicology in the Tropics.* London. Taylor and Francis. 1980.

Not the title of a torrid romance, this book is in 4 parts, "the first deals with links between the occurrence of toxic substances in the tropical environment and certain human diseases. The second section is concerned with chemical carcinogens which can contaminate foodstuffs, e.g., aflatoxins and N-nitroso compounds. The third part provides an overview of several groups of compounds including drugs, alkaloids, cyanogenic glycosides and pesticides. The last section is concerned with risk-benefit assessment of drugs and inter-ethnic differences in responses to and disposition of drugs.''

143. Tsubaki T, Irukayama K, eds. *Minamata Disease: Methylmercury Poisoning in Minamata and Niigata, Japan.* Tokyo. Kodansha, Ltd. 1977.

A scientific survey of the 1953 methylmercury poisoning epidemic in Japan. Includes historical and background information, pathology and clinical aspects of the disease, and countermeasures. An appendix discusses methylmercury concentration in the Agano River.

144. Vershueren K. *Handbook of Environmental Data on Organic Chemicals.* New York. Van Nostrand Reinhold Company. 1977.

Data presented on more than 1000 chemicals includes chemical and physical properties, information on air pollution and water pollution, and biological effects of organisms from microorganisms to man. 347 references used in compiling this handbook.

145. Waldbott GL. *Health Effects of Environmental Pollutants.* St. Louis, MO. Mosby. 1978.

In 25 chapters, this textbook covers sources of pollutants, including their dispersion in the environment. Chemical agents, radiation, smoking, water and noise pollution, and fire are among the subjects treated. Glossary, author, and subject indexes.

See also:

Gelboin HV. *Genetic and Environmental Factors in Experimental and Human Cancer.* [under *Carcinogenesis, Mutagenesis, Teratogenesis*]

Getz ME. *Paper and Thin-Layer Chromatographic Analysis of Environmental Toxicants.* [under *Analytical Toxicology*]

Guthrie FE. *Introduction to Environmental Toxicology.* [under *General Textbooks*]

Khan MAQ. *Pesticide and Xenobiotic Metabolism in Aquatic Organisms.* [under *Pesticides*]

Purdom PW. *Environmental Health.* [under *General Textbooks*]

Strik JJTWA. *Chemical Porphyria in Man.* [under *Target Systems*]

Section on *Occupational Health and Industrial Hygiene*

Section on *Pesticides*

Section on *Physical Hazards*

Chapter on *Special Monographs*

Food

146. Boyd E. *Toxicity of Pure Foods*. Cleveland. CRC Press. 1973.

Presents "recent evidence on the toxicity of pure foods, carbohydrates, fats, proteins, salts, water, vitamins, and food adjuvants such as caffeine." Food additives and contaminants are not within the scope of this book.

147. Connors CK. *Food Additives and Hyperactive Children*. New York. Plenum Press. 1980.

Discusses behavioral and learning disorders of children, and their relationship to food additives. Numerous clinical trials are cited. Two of the appendices are a "Hyperkinesis Study Diet" and a "Cytotoxic Food Test."

148. Food Safety Council. Scientific Committee. *Proposed System for Food Safety Assessment*. In *Food and Cosmetics Toxicology* 16(Suppl 2) Dec. 1978. Oxford. Pergamon Press.

The task of the committee preparing this report was "to search out and study the world's body of knowledge regarding food safety testing and to recommend new criteria by which a comprehensive assessment of risk could be determined."

149. Furia TE, ed. *Handbook of Food Additives*, 2nd ed. Cleveland. CRC Press. Volume 1-1972, Volume 2-1980.

Color additives, sweeteners, phosphates, gums, acidulants, antioxidants, vitamins, and enzymes are among the substances to which separate chapters have been devoted. Thousands of references. A concluding chapter on the "Regulatory Status of Direct Food Additives" presents in tabular form food additives and their synonyms, the Flavor Extract Manufacturer's Association Number, the regulation affecting the substance, and limitations.

150. Galli CL, Paoleti R, Vettorazzi G, eds. *Chemical Toxicology of Food*. Amsterdam. Elsevier/North-Holland. 1978.

Proceedings of an international symposium held in Milan. Volume 3 of the series *Developments in Toxicology and Environmental Science*. The program presents "views on the evaluation of toxicological aspects of food additives, at both the biological and technological levels. The current legislation and its implications for the changing patterns in food toxicology in different countries have also been discussed in considerable detail.'' Topics such as risk-benefit, acceptable daily intake, regulatory issues, reproductive toxicology, and allergic responses are among those included.

151. Hui YH. *United States Food Laws, Regulations, and Standards.* New York. John Wiley and Sons. 1979.

A fine distillation of the major legislation, regulations and standards applying to food in this country. Arranged by the agencies most directly dealing with food—Department of Agriculture, Department of Commerce, CPSC, EPA, FTC, FDA, and the Bureau of Alcohol, Tobacco and Firearms of the Department of Treasury. Numerous standards have been paraphrased or reprinted by the author.

152. Leonard BJ. *Toxicological Aspects of Food Safety.* In *Archives of Toxicology* (Suppl 1) Berlin. Springer-Verlag. 1978.

Proceedings of the European Society of Toxicology Meeting held in Copenhagen in June, 1977. The papers provide detailed accounts of various aspects of food safety and toxicity.

153. Leung AY. *Encyclopedia of Common Natural Ingredients: Used in Food, Drugs, and Cosmetics.* New York. John Wiley. 1980.

Information on natural ingredients—names and synonyms, physical description, chemical composition, biological activity, pharmacology, uses, commercial preparations, and regulatory status.

154. Liener IE, ed. *Toxic Constituents of Plant Foodstuffs,* 2nd ed. New York. Academic Press. 1980.

A volume in the monographic series *Food Science and Technology,* this book should be of current interest because of the increasing use of plant protein in the human diet. Chapters cover the following natural food constituents—protease inhibitors, hemagglutins, glucosinolates, cyanogens, saponins, gossypol lathyrogens. Other topics include favism, allergens, carcinogens and processing as a toxicity inducer. There is even a section on flatulence as produced by legumes and other foods.

155. National Research Council. Food and Nutrition Board. Committee on Food Protection. *Toxicants Occurring Naturally in Foods,* 2nd ed. Washington, DC. National Academy of Sciences. 1973.

Covering substances that are natural components in foods and not intentional or accidental additives. Separately authored chapters on trace elements, toxic proteins and peptides, food lipids, antivitamins, oxalates, seafood toxicants, etc. The final chapter offers an overview on the "toxicology of natural food chemicals," discusses risks, safety benefits and compares normal components of food with food contaminants.

156. US Congress. Office of Technology Assessment. *Environmental Contaminants in Food*. Washington, DC. US Congress. Office of Technology Assessment. 1979.

"The assessment is concerned with chemical and radioactive contaminants that inadvertently find their way into the human food supply." Looks at federal and state laws and regulations, methods for assessing health risks, regulatory decisionmaking, monitoring and instrumentation, and congressional options. Numerous tables. Interesting appendices including "Substances Whose Production or Environmental Release are Likely to Increase in the next 10 years," "Measuring Benefits and Costs," and "Analysis of Foods for Radioactivity".

See also:

Miller EC. *Naturally Occurring Carcinogens-Mutagens and Modulators of Carcinogensis*. [under *Carcinogenesis, Mutagenesis, Teratogenesis*]

Legislative, Regulatory, and Societal Issues

157. Coulston F, ed. *Regulatory Aspects of Carcinogenesis and Food Additives: the Delaney Clause*. New York. Academic Press. 1979.

Volume 2 in the series *Ecotoxicology and Environmental Quality*. The regulation of carcinogenic food additives is the focus of papers in this volume. Much discussion of impact of the Delaney clause, regulation, extrapolation, and decision making.

158. Dominguez G, ed. *Guidebook: Toxic Substances Control Act*. Cleveland. CRC Press. 1977.

Includes the complete text of TOSCA. A guidebook for the chemical industry, an aid to interpretation of and compliance with TOSCA, its effects in terms of costs, management, testing. Large list of environmental and toxicological testing laboratories organized by state and country which contains names, addresses, testing done, classes of compounds studies, capabilities available and personnel employed.

159. *Environmental Law Handbook,* 6th ed. Washington, DC. Government Institutes. 1979.

A leading reference book in environmental legislation. An introductory chapter serves as either a law primer or review, covering the court system and briefly describing concepts such as torts, negligence, constitutional laws, defenses, evidence, and liability. The remainder of the book covers broad areas of environmental concern and discusses pertinent legislation in each of these areas. There are chapters on the National Environmental Policy Act, water pollution control, air pollution control, land use, pesticides, toxic substances, noise, and solid and hazardous wastes. State and local, in addition to federal, governmental policy is discussed. Specific cases are included as examples.

160. *Environmental Statutes.* Washington, DC. Government Institutes. 1980.

Contains the texts of the following laws: Clear Air Act, Federal Water Pollution Control Act, Clean Water Act of 1977, National Environmental Policy Act, Noise Control Act, Occupational Safety and Health Act, Resource Conservation and Recovery Act, Safe Drinking Water Act, Toxic Substances Control Act.

161. Frick WG, ed. *Environmental Glossary.* Washington, DC. Government Institutes. 1980.

This compilation of definitions is drawn primarily from environmental legislation and the *Code of Federal Regulations.* Each definition is keyed to the particular source from which it is taken. Additional terms have been defined based on unpublished EPA documents.

162. McRae A, Whelchel L, eds. *Toxic Substances Control Sourcebook.* Germantown, MD. Aspen Systems. 1978.

A discussion of toxic substance regulation and compliance intended to guide "decision-makers through the complexities of law, implementation, compliance and effective management." Substantial space devoted to impact on industry with a chapter devoted to "significant cases involving toxic substances." A group of appendices includes full texts or excerpts of important acts.

163. Mendeloff J. *Regulating Safety: An Economic and Political Analysis of Occupational Safety and Health Policy.* Cambridge. MIT Press. 1979.

Covers important economic and political issues spawned as a result of OSHA. Topics such as standard setting, enforcement, effectiveness, and OSHA's safety program are analyzed.

164. Miller ML, ed. *Toxic Control in the 80's.* Washington, DC. Government Institutes. 1980.

Volume 4 of the *Toxic Control Series,* this publication consists of proceedings of the 4th Toxic Control Conference held in Washington, DC on December 10-11, 1979. Papers on TOSCA, OSHA, RCRA, good laboratory practice, premanufacture notification, a national cancer policy, small companies, the superfund issue, hazardous wastes, confidentiality, multilateral trade negotiations, etc.

165. Northrup HR, Rowan RL, Perry CR. *The Impact of OSHA.* Philadelphia. Industrial Research Unit, the Wharton School, University of Pennsylvania. 1978.

Number 17 in the series, *Labor Relations and Public Policy.* Consists of details on and results of four studies: two industry studies—on the aerospace and chemical industries and two hazard studies—on vinyl chloride and cotton/dust noise in the textile industry.

166. Ross S, Pronin M, eds. *Toxic Substances Sourcebook.* New York. Environment Information Center. 1978.

Most of this book is devoted to abstracts of recent literature. Also, list of periodicals, books, films, data bases. Discussion of regulations with extracts from the *Federal Register.* Emphasis on TOSCA.

167. *Toxic Substances Sourcebook 2.* New York. Environment Information Center. 1980.

Volume 2 of EIC's Toxic Substances Sourcebook Series is again devoted primarily to abstracts of journal articles. Valuable preliminary material on risk assessment, TSCA, OSHA, NIOSH, legislation and regulations. Lists of conferences, books, films, and periodicals.

168. Vettorazzi G. *International Regulatory Aspects for Pesticide Chemicals.* Boca Raton, FL. CRC Press. 1979.

A joint Food and Agriculture Organization and World Health Organization statement of the toxicologic evaluation of pesticides. Profiles are provided for some 130 chemicals, with such data as uses, metabolism, toxicology, no-effect levels, and residues.

See also:

Epstein S. *The Politics of Cancer.* [under *Carcinogenesis, Mutagenesis, Teratogenesis*]

Hui YH. *United States Food Laws, Regulations, and Standards.* [under *Food*]

Occupational Exposure Guide. [under *Occupational Health and Industrial Hygiene*]

Peters GA. *Sourcebook on Asbestos Diseases.* [under *Environmental Toxicology*]

Tedeschi CG. *Forensic Medicine.* [under *Clinical Toxicology*]

Metals

169. Berman E. *Toxic Metals and Their Analysis*. London. Heydon. 1980.

Individual toxic metals and metalloids are discussed in 31 chapters, the metals' toxicology, bodily distribution, dietary concentrations, and methods of analysis are covered. Among the analytical methods discussed are colorimetry, fluorimetry, chromatography, polarography, and spectroscopy.

170. Commission of the European Communities. *Criteria (Dose/Effect Relationships) for Cadmium*. Oxford. Pergamon Press. 1978.

Properties, occurrence, environmental concentrations, metabolism, toxicology.

171. Friberg L, Magnus P, Nordberg GF, Kjellstrom T. *Cadmium in the Environment*. Cleveland. CRC Press. 1974.

"... focuses upon information essential to the understanding of the toxic action of cadmium and the relationship between exposure and effects on human beings and animals." One chapter of interest concentrates on cadmium in Japan and its epidemiological aspects in regard to Itai-itai disease, and on cadmium pollution in various areas of Japan.

172. Friberg L, Nordberg GF, Vouk VB, eds. *Handbook on the Toxicology of Metals*. Amsterdam. Elsevier. 1979.

Biological/toxic effects of metals in man. Part 1 discusses general aspects of metals such as chemistry, analysis, transport in the environment, routes of exposure, effects, prevention of poisoning, diagnosis and treatment, mutagenicity and carcinogenicity. Part 2 consists of chapters devoted to specific metals. Metal chapters organized consistently with abstract, physical and chemical properties, methods and problems of analysis, production and uses, environmental levels and exposures, metabolism, levels in tissues and biological fluids, effects and dose-response relationships. A complete and well documented text on this important subject.

173. Friberg L, Vostal J, eds. *Mercury in the Environment: An Epidemiological and Toxicological Appraisal*. Cleveland. CRC Press. 1972.

A major review on the toxicity of mercury. Analytical methods, transport, environmental transformation, metabolism, clinical signs of intoxication, are all treated in detail. Additional topics are mercury in human tissue and urine, inorganic mercury, organic mercury compounds, and genetic effects.

174. Goyer RA, Mehlman MA, eds. *Toxicology of Trace Elements*. Washington, DC. Hemisphere Publishing Company. 1977.

Volume 2 of *Advance in Modern Toxicology*. Toxic effects of mercury, lead, arsenic, copper, nickel, vanadium, and tellurium are emphasized. Additional discussion of nutrient interactions with toxic elements, and metal carcinogenesis.

175. Kharasch N, ed. *Trace Metals in Health and Disease*. New York. Raven Press. 1979.

"Topics ranging from new aspects of the impact of metals in the environment on human health to the roles of metals in genetic information transfer are discussed. Particular attention is focused on the role of metals in carcinogenesis, and the possible role of metal-induced mutagenesis in the initiation of cancer is explored."

176. Luckey TD, Venugopal B. *Metal Toxicity in Mammals*. New York. Plenum Press. 1977.

Volume 1 "Physiologic and Chemical Basis for Metal Toxicity." Volume 2 "Chemical Toxicity of Metals and Metalloids." Volume 1 includes such topics as intake, absorption, detoxication, excretion, physico-chemical properties, carcinogenicity/teratogenicity. Chapter 6 of this volume offers a summary and overview of metal toxicity arranged by groups and subgroups and makes generalizations about these categories where possible.

177. Mennear JH, ed. *Cadmium Toxicity*. New York. Marcel Dekker. 1979.

Volume 15 of the series *Modern Pharmacology—Toxicology*. Six chapters centered on the manner in which cadmium influences mammalian systems plus one on environmental flow of cadmium in the US and one on analytical methods.

178. National Research Council. Committee on Lead in the Human Environment. *Lead in the Human Environment*. Washington, DC. National Academy of Sciences. 1980.

This report is similar in format to those issued by the former Committee on Medical and Biologic Effects of Environmental Pollutants of the National Research Council (see *Special Monographs*). It has been prepared by an expert committee and offers "a systematic approach to making decisions about lead in the human environment". Regulatory issues are discussed as well.

179. Needleman HL, ed. *Low Level Lead Exposure: The Clinical Implications of Current Research*. New York. Raven Press. 1980.

In 24 papers, the problems of low level lead exposure are examined in population and animal studies, as well as from the public health, economic, and regulatory perspectives. Two papers discuss the Massachusetts Childhood Lead-Poisoning Prevention Program.

180. Oehme FW, ed. *Toxicity of Heavy Metals in the Environment.* New York. Marcel Dekker. 1978.

Volume 2 of the series *Hazardous and Toxic Substances.* "This book has been organized by first discussing the basic concepts and principles of heavy metal pollution, how the heavy metals enter the environment and animal or human food chain, and the fundamental principles and mechanisms of toxicity due to heavy metal chemicals." Individual metals, trace heavy metals, and metallic compounds are then discussed along with concluding chapters on quantitative assays and chelation therapy.

181. Sigel H, ed. *Carcinogenicity and Metal Ions.* New York. Marcel Dekker. 1980.

Volume 10 of the series *Metal Ions in Biological Systems.* Among the topics in this volume are metals and tumor development, metal ions in malignant tissue development, trace element and human leukemia, zinc and cyancobalamin in tumor growth.

182. Singhal RL, Thomas JA, eds. *Lead Toxicity.* Baltimore. Urban and Schwarzenberg. 1980.

A compendium of reviews of recent advances in lead toxicity research. Chapters on lead and neurotoxicity, the kidney, energy metabolism, heme biosynthesis, neurophysiological effects, human exposure, etc. Other interesting chapters include "Nutrient-lead interactions" and "Chronic effects of lead in nonhuman primates."

183. Tsuchiya K, ed. *Cadmium Studies in Japan: A Review.* Amsterdam. Elsevier/North Holland. 1978.

Covers experimental and etiologic studies on cadmium toxicity with an emphasis on the etiology of "itai-itai" disease. Administrative studies of 12 district prefectures.

184. Webb M, ed. *The Chemistry, Biochemistry, and Biology of Cadmium.* Amsterdam. Elsevier/North-Holland. 1979.

A complete monographic review of the metal cadmium. Chapters on cadmium in soils and vegetation, in aquatic organisms, intracellular effects, mammalian distribution, metallothioneins, biological effects in mammals, toxicology of cadmium-thionein, cadmium in man, etc.

See also:

Gomez M. *At Work in Copper.* [under *Occupational Health*]

Tsubaki T. *Minamata Disease.* [under *Environmental Toxicology*]

Chapter on *Special Monographs*

Occupational Health and Industrial Hygiene

185. American Conference of Governmental Industrial Hygienists. Committee on Threshold Limit Values. *Documentation of the Threshold Limit Values for Substances in Workroom Air,* 4th ed. Cincinnati. American Conference of Governmental Industrial Hygienists. 1980.

This publication provides the scientific information and data which are used to determine threshold limit values.

186. Browning E. *Toxicity and Metabolism of Industrial Solvents.* Amsterdam. Elsevier. 1965.

Still the most complete compilation of data relating to the toxicity and metabolism of solvents—hydrocarbons, alcohols, ketones, acetals, ethers, esters, glycols, silicium compounds and other assorted compounds. References for all data cited.

187. Cohen EN. *Anesthetic Exposure in the Workplace.* Littleton, MA. PSG Publishing Company. 1980.

Anesthetic gases are considered from the viewpoint of constituting a potential occupational hazard to physicians and various allied medical professions. After a brief historical chapter, the book examines this hazard to humans and animals, further investigates mechanisms of toxicity and control methods, and concludes with chapters on the role of the government and medical/legal implications, especially in relation to NIOSH and OSHA.

188. *Encyclopaedia of Occupational Health and Safety.* Geneva. International Labour Office. 1971.

In 2 volumes, a practical encyclopedia, concentrating on risks and preventive measures. Contributions from 70 countries. Authors and their countries are identified for each entry. References.

189. Frazier CA, ed. *Occupational Asthma.* New York. Van Nostrand Reinhold. 1980.

Chapters on meatwrapper's asthma, baker's asthma, hoya (sea-squirt) asthma, asthma caused by western red cedar, wood dust, vinyl chloride, pharmacologic dusts, castor-bean dust, fumes from pine rosin and epoxy rosin systems. Byssinosis, pneumoconiosis, bagassosis, and asthma in laboratory animal workers are also considered.

190. Gardner AW, ed. *Current Approaches to Occupational Medicine.* Bristol. John Wright. 1979.

Reviews on miscellaneous topics such as lead, gases, asbestos, fibres, toxicity testing, epidemiology, food hygiene, alcohol, stress, and shift work.

191. Gomez M, Duffy R, Trivelli V. *At Work in Copper: Occupational Health and Safety in Copper Smelting.* New York. INFORM. 1979.

A detailed 3 volume study on potential hazards in the copper industry. Of interest not only to the copper industry but to those concerned with industrial health and safety generally and its interaction with regulatory agencies. INFORM provides ratings for various aspects of specific, named copper plants. Senator Harrison Williams' preface states, "This study will give the public a rare look into the working conditions in copper smelters and the health problems smelter workers face.... This INFORM project will generate a vigorous public interest in the health and safety conditions in our nation's factories, mills, shops and foundries."

192. Hamilton A. *Industrial Toxicology,* 4th ed. Acton, MA. Publishing Sciences Group. 1974.

Concentrates on occupational diseases. Substantial chapters on over 36 metals. Chemical compounds, radiation, dusts, and biological hazards are discussed. Extensive bibliography and a glossary of occupational medicine terms.

193. Hughes JP, Proctor NH, eds. *Chemical Hazards of the Workplace.* Philadelphia. Lippincott. 1978.

Initial chapters on evaluation of hazards and occupational disease followed by a guide to chemical hazards. Describes "the potential effects of exposure to those 400 or so toxic substances likely to be encountered at work ... presents the fundamentals of toxicology for each chemical, lists the clinical signs of overexposure, identifies the medical measures most successful in the early detection of adverse effects, and suggests accepted methods of treatment."

194. Hunter D. *The Diseases of Occupations,* 6th ed. London. Hodder and Stoughton. 1978.

A very large and readable monograph that reviews "disease in relation to occupation." The author is a physician and the perspective clinical. Unusual is its strong historical orientation which gives us insights into the similarities and differences between occupational safety and health today and its origins. Chapters concentrating on individual chemicals, noxious gases, skin and cancer diseases, physical agents, pneumoconioses, accidents, etc. Indexed and with many illustrations.

195. Key MM, Henschel AF, Butler J, Ligo RN, Tabershaw IR, eds. *Occupational Diseases: A Guide to Their Recognition,* revised ed. Washington,

DC. US Department of Health, Education and Welfare, Public Health Service, Center for Disease Control, National Institute for Occupational Safety and Health. 1977.

A manual meant to aid in the identification of occupational diseases. Chapters focus on routes of entry and mechanisms of action, infectious diseases, skin diseases, airway diseases, plant poisoning, chemical hazards, pesticides, carcinogens, and physical hazards. A concluding section on sources of consultation and reference aids in the occupational health field.

196. Lemen R, Dement JM, eds. *Dusts and Disease.* Park Forest South, IL. Pathotox. 1979.

Consists of the proceedings of the Conference on Occupational Exposures to Fibrous and Particulate Dust and their Extension into the Environment. Papers presented in eight sessions devoted to topics such as fiber pathogenicity, asbestos, mineral-contaminated talc, nonfibrous talc, inorganic synthetic fibers, nonfibrous particulates, and government response. Conference co-sponsored by the Society for Occupational and Environmental Health and the Mine Safety and Health Administration.

197. Linch AL. *Biological Monitoring for Industrial Chemical Exposure Control.* Cleveland. CRC Press. 1974.

Starting with the premise that man himself is the best indicator of his workplace environment, the author devotes careful attention to urine, blood, and breath analysis. Physiological monitoring of bodily systems, biological threshold limits, and quality control in sampling and laboratory analysis are other topics covered.

198. Mackison FW, Stricoff RS, Partridge LJ Jr, eds. *NIOSH/OSHA Pocket Guide to Chemical Hazards.* Cincinnati. National Institute of Occupational Safety and Health. 1978.

''. . . presents, in tabular form, information and recommendations relating to permissible exposure limits, chemical and physical properties, health hazard information, respiratory protection, and personal protection and sanitation practices for 380 specific chemicals for which there are Federal regulations.''

199. McCann M. *Artist Beware.* New York. Watson-Guptill Publications. 1979.

A fascinating account of and practical guide to the hazards of art-related professions. Part 1 examines various art materials and how they affect body organs and systems, plus considering studio safety, ventilation, and protective devices. Part 2 is devoted to the hazards of specific procedures such as painting, printmaking, sculpture, metalworking, and photography.

200. Monson RR. *Occupational Epidemiology.* CRC Press. Boca Raton, FL. 1980.

> A chapter on the history of epidemiology covering such key individuals as John Graunt, William Farr, and John Snow and including the Doll and Hill cigarette studies, is followed by chapters which generally review epidemiologic methodology such as the nature, collection, analysis and interpretation of epidemiologic data. The remainder of the book is devoted to occupational epidemiology and discusses studies of morbidity and mortality, surveys of the health status of the employed, and other current problems in occupational epidemiology. Brief glossary of terms.

201. National Research Council. *Prudent Practices for Handling Hazardous Chemicals in Laboratories.* Washington, DC. National Academy Press. 1981.

> Offers guidelines for the safe handling of chemicals in laboratories. Physical hazards (such as fire, explosion, electric shock, cuts) are covered as well as acute and chronic chemical hazards. Laboratory ventilation (e.g. hoods), protective equipment such as glasses and gloves, storage cabinets, and disposal methods are other topics considered.

202. *Occupational Exposure Guide.* Neenah, WI. JJ Keller and Associates. 1979.

> This loose-leaf publication consists primarily of a compendium of OSHA regulations. Includes lists of state plans, OSHA field locations, sources of consultation. This is part of Keller's *Hazardous Substances Guide Series.* Other titles in the series include *Hazardous Substances Advisor, Hazardous Materials Guide, Toxic Substances Guide,* and *Pesticides Guide.* The focus in each of these is on compliance and regulatory activity.

203. *Patty's Industrial Hygiene and Toxicology,* 3rd revised ed. New York. Wiley. Volume I "General Principles," 1978; Volume II "Toxicology," 1980; Volume III "Theory and Rationale of Industrial Hygiene Practice," 1979. Various editors.

> A giant compendium of immeasurable reference value, these volumes are among the most complete sources for occupational health information.

204. Peterson JE. *Industrial Health.* Englewood Cliffs, NJ. Prentice-Hall. 1977.

> Covering all the salient principles yet requiring only a minimum of scientific background, this book provides a solid introduction to industrial health. In addition to chemicals, areas such as abnormal pressure,

noise, biothermal stress, and radiation are treated. Appendices contain a review of organic chemical nomenclature and a glossary.

205. Plunkett ER. *Handbook of Industrial Toxicology,* 2nd ed. New York. Chemical Publishing Company. 1976.

> A handbook of chemicals. Entries for each substance include descriptive data, occupational exposures, threshold limit values, toxicities, and preventive measures.

206. Plunkett ER. *Occupational Diseases: A Syllabus of Signs and Symptoms.* Stamford, CT. Barrett Book Company. 1977.

> "A quick reference source for aid in evaluating the occupational cause of a particular symptom." The bulk of the book alphabetically lists symptoms, occupational groups which may be affected (according to Ramazzini) and possible causes. Another list alphabetically lists toxins and presents symptoms associated with each. Includes a list of common names for occupational diseases (e.g., carpet layer's knee = prepatellar bursitis).

207. Proctor NH, Hughes JP. *Chemical Hazards of the Workplace.* Philadelphia. JB Lippincott. 1978.

> A handbook for the occupational physician dealing with patient care. Introductory chapters on toxicologic concepts, hazard evaluation, environmental control, occupational disease diagnosis and treatment, and chemically induced pulmonary disease. Remainder of book consists of monographs on 386 chemical substances. Entries on nomenclature, physical form of substance, uses, means of exposure, toxicology, treatment, and medical control.

208. Sax NI. *Dangerous Properties of Industrial Materials,* 5th ed. New York. Van Nostrand Reinhold. 1979.

> 12 sections, each written by an expert in the field. "General Chemicals" section provides a single source for quick, up-to-date concise hazard-analysis information for nearly 15,000 common industrial laboratory materials." Radiation, noise and fire, and solid waste treatment hazards and equipment for control are discussed. There is a section on requirements for labeling and identification of hazardous materials. ACGIH TLV's for 1978 are included. The book considers not just "industrial materials" but the entire industrial environment. "Addendum of very newly listed carcinogens, neoplastigens."

209. US Congress. House Committee on Education and Labor. Subcommittee on Labor Standards. *Occupational Diseases and Their Compensation.*

Hearings, 96th Congress, First Session. Washington, DC. US Government Printing Office. 1980.

Part 1 discusses asbestos and its diseases and part 2 discusses other toxics. Provocative testimony, statements, and attachments aimed at examining the entire problem of work-related disease and manner of compensation.

210. Xintaras C, Johnson BL, de Groot I, eds. *Behavioral Toxicology: Early Detection of Occupational Hazards.* Washington, DC. US Department of Health, Education and Welfare, Public Health Service, Center for Disease Control, National Institute for Occupational Safety and Health. 1974.

Consists of Proceedings of a Behavioral Toxicology Workshop. Sessions devoted to workplace exposure to pesticides, solvents, metals, gases, irritants, odors, etc. Workshop demonstrations consisting of test batteries for various exposures are also presented along with illustrative photographs.

211. Zenz C, ed. *Developments in Occupational Medicine.* Chicago. Year Book Medical Publishers. 1980.

A continuation of *Occupational Medicine: Principles and Practical Applications,* also edited by Carl Zenz. Twenty expert contributors investigate epidemiology, working women, the physical working environment, and the psychosocial and chemical working environments. There are chapters on reproductive toxicology, ergonomics, occupational stress, solvent-related disorders, and pesticides, among others. An appendix provides "A summary of NIOSH Recommendations for Occupational Health Standards".

See also:

De Bruin A. *Biochemical Toxicology of Environmental Agents.* [under *Environmental Toxicology*]

Fouts JR, ed. *Industrial and Environmental Xenobiotics: In vitro versus in vivo Biotransformation and Toxicity.* [under *Environmental Toxicology*]

Mendeloff J. *Regulating Safety.* [under *Legislative, Regulatory, and Societal Issues*]

Parkes WR. *Occupational Lung Diseases.* [under *Target Systems*]

Preger L, ed. *Induced Disease: Drug, Irradiation, Occupation.* [under *Drugs*]

Shaw CR, ed. Prevention of Occupational Cancer. [under *Carcinogenesis, Mutagenesis, Teratogenesis*]

Pesticides

212. Brooks GT. *Chlorinated Insecticides.* Cleveland. CRC Press. 1974.

In two volumes (I-Technology and Application, II-Biological and Environmental Aspects), an authoritative work on chlorinated insecticides.

213. Brown AWA. *Ecology of Pesticides.* New York. John Wiley. 1978.

Includes topics such as the effects of insecticides on plants, arthropid fauna, soil invertebrates and microflora, aquatic invertebrate biota, fish, terrestrial vertebrates, and birds. Organochlorine insecticides and eggshell thinning and insecticide residues are other topics of interest. Additional chapters on herbicides and fungicides in the ecosystem.

214. Caswell RL, ed. *Pesticide Handbook, 1979–80,* 28th ed. College Park, MD. Entomological Society of America. 1979.

Includes a large variety of information, tables, statistics. Data on rates of application, analytical toxicology labs, EPA regional contacts, applications and limitations on classes of pesticides, pesticides and the environment, regulatory documents, cancelled and suspended pesticides, lists of product names and ingredients, and sources of additional information.

215. Edwards CA. *Persistent Pesticides in the Environment,* 2nd ed. Cleveland. CRC Press. 1973.

A review of the literature on pesticidal residues in the environment. Both the physical environment and biological organisms are discussed.

216. Eto M. *Organophosphorus Pesticides: Organic and Biological Chemistry.* Cleveland. CRC Press. 1974.

Structure, synthesis, chemical reactions and biochemistry of organophosphorus pesticides are covered. Attention is also paid to specific pesticides. Information included on selective toxicity, chemical interactions, and side effects.

217. *Farm Chemicals Handbook 1980.* Willoughby, OH. Meister Publishing. 1980.

The major portion of this yearbook is a pesticide dictionary which ''is a compilation of experimental and commercial pesticides available in the US and around the world.'' Among the data for each pesticide are actions, applications, formulations, and toxicity.

218. Hart RW, ed. *A Rational Evaluation of Pesticidal vs. Mutagenic/Carcinogenic Action.* Bethesda, MD. US Department of Health, Education, and Welfare, Public Health Service, National Institutes of Health. 1978. [DHEW Publication # (NIH) 78-1306]

This book developed from a 1976 eponymic conference. Part 1 on chemical evaluation includes chapters on structure-activity relationships of antischistosomals and the evaluation of environmentally safe pesticides. Part 2 on biological evaluations covers mutagenicity assays, cytogenetic effects, and use of DNA damage as a prescreen for carcinogenesis/mutagenesis.

219. Hayes WJ. *Toxicology of Pesticides,* 3rd revised ed. Baltimore. Williams and Wilkins. 1975.

". . . deals with the principles, the general conditions of exposure, the observed effects of this exposure on human health, the problems of diagnosis and treatment, the means of preventing injury, and brief outlines of the impact of pesticides on domestic animals and wildlife." CAS registry numbers and chemical names for all compounds mentioned in text.

220. *Herbicide Handbook of the Weed Science Society of America, 4th ed.* Champaign, IL, Weed Science Society of America. 1979.

Alphabetical listing of herbicides. Provides information on nomenclature and properties, herbicidal use, use precautions, physiological and biochemical behavior, behavior in soils, toxicology (includes acute, subacute, chronic toxicities, general toxicity to wildlife and fish, skin toxicity, poisoning symptoms, first aid and antidotes), analytical methods and synthesis, and references.

221. Khan MAQ, Lech JJ, Menn JJ, eds. *Pesticide and Xenobiotic Metabolism in Aquatic Organisms.* Washington, DC. American Chemical Society. 1979.

Based on a symposium sponsored by the Division of Pesticide Chemistry at the 176th Meeting of the American Chemical Society, Miami Beach, Florida, September 11–17, 1978. Number 99 in the *ACS Symposium Series.* Concerned with the relatively young area of research in biotransformation of xenobiotics in fish and other aquatic organisms. Among the organisms covered are Japanese carp, mosquitofish, dogfish shark, and rainbow trout. Chemicals studied include organophosphorous insecticides, PCBs, pentachlorophenol, aromatic hydrocarbons, and petroleum hydrocarbons.

222. Kuhr RJ, Dorough HW. *Carbamate Insecticides: Chemistry, Biochemistry, and Toxicology.* Cleveland. CRC Press. 1976.

The authors have done credit to carbamates as one of the major insecticide classes by preparing a thorough review of their chemistry, mode of action, toxicology, metabolism, and environmental effects.

223. Martin H, Worthing CR, eds. *Pesticide Manual: Basic Information on the Chemicals Used as Active Components of Pesticides*. London. British Crop Protection Council. 1974.

Technical information on the active ingredients of pesticides used in agriculture.

224. Matsumura F. *Toxicology of Insecticides*. New York. Plenum Press. 1975.

Designed as a text for "graduate students and the general scientific community rather than those already expert in the field," this book covers general principles and treats specific insecticides and classes of insecticides plus metabolism, entry into animal and environmental systems, the hazards to man and domestic animals.

225. White-Stevens R, ed. *Pesticides in the Environment,* multi-volume. New York. Marcel Dekker. 1976.

Covers chemistry, biology, metabolism of pesticides, their analysis, residues, toxicology, pest resistance, their role in crop protection, management of forests and preservation.

226. Wilkinson CF, ed. *Insecticide Biochemistry and Physiology*. New York. Plenum Press. 1976.

A complete discussion of the mode of action of insecticides in 5 parts: 1. "Penetration and Distribution," 2. "Metabolism," 3. "Target Site Interaction," 4. "Selectivity and Resistance," and 5. "Insecticide Toxicology." Among the specific areas covered are enzymatic conjugation, acetylcholinesterase inhibition and nervous system effects, other chronic effects such as cancer, insecticide interactions, treatment of poisoning, and environmental toxicology. A chemical index lists substances used in the text alphabetically by common name and identifies chemical name and structure with each.

See also:

Brown VK. *Acute Toxicity in Theory and Practice.* [under *Clinical Toxicology*]

Cattabeni F. *Dioxin: Toxicological and Chemical Aspects.* [under *Environmental Toxicology*]

Vettorazzi G. *International Regulatory Aspects for Pesticide Chemicals.* [under *Legislative, Regulatory, and Societal Issues*]

Section on *Environmental Toxicology*

Physical Hazards

227. Assenheim HM, ed. *Biological Effects of Radio-Frequency and Microwave Radiation.* Ottawa. National Research Council Canada, Associate Committee on Scientific Criteria for Environmental Quality. 1979.

Summarizes worldwide research on microwave and radio-frequency radiation. Discusses physical principles and biological effects (including epidemiology and exposure standard criteria).

228. Baranski, Czerski P. *Biological Effects of Microwaves.* Stroudsbourg, PA. Dowden, Hutchinson, and Ross. 1976.

"A survey of the literature on the biological effects of microwaves, including the available data on evaluation of health hazards and safe exposure limits."

229. Hall EJ. *Radiobiology for the Radiologist,* 2nd ed. Hagerstown, MD. Harper and Row. 1978.

A good introductory text on the effects of radiation on cells, tissues, biological systems. Includes chapters on carcinogenesis, genetic changes, effects on embryo and fetus, and risk benefit.

230. Henderson D, Hamernik RP, Dosanjh DS, Mills JH, eds. *Effects of Noise on Hearing.* New York. Raven Press. 1976.

"Useful as a text and sourcebook for audiologists, otolaryngologists, engineers, sensory psychologists, and environmental scientists". Covers cochlear anatomy/biochemistry, electrophysiological/mechanical features of the ear, experimental, epidemiological. and analytical studies of noise-induced hearing loss, and bases for establishing a damage risk criteria.

231. May DN, ed. *Handbook of Noise Assessment.* New York. Van Nostrand Reinhold. 1978.

This discussion of noise assessment examines both psychological and physical effects. Chapters devoted to noise of surface transportation, air transportation, recreational vehicles, hospitals, industrial sites, commercial sites, the home, etc. Appendices on acoustical standards and regulating agencies plus a glossary.

232. Michaelson SM, Miller MW, Magin R, Carstensen EL, eds. *Fundamental and Applied Aspects of Nonionizing Radiation.* New York. Plenum Press. 1975.

Consists of the proceedings of the 7th Rochester International Conference on Environmental Toxicity. Papers presented on biophysics, energy absorption, biological effects of microwaves and ultrasound, medical applications, and occupational aspects.

233. National Research Council. *Considerations of Health Benefit-Cost Analysis for Activities Involving Ionizing Radiation Exposure and Alternatives.* Washington, DC. National Academy of Sciences. 1977.

An analytical approach covering concepts of cost-benefit analysis, including legal aspects. Analyses for medical radiation and energy production are discussed.

234. National Research Council. Advisory Committee on the Biological Effects of Ionizing Radiation. *The Effects on Populations of Exposure to Low Levels of Ionizing Radiation.* Washington, DC. National Academy of Sciences. 1972.

A classic report that deals with the scientific basis for the establishment of radiation protection standards and encompasses a review and reevaluation of existing scientific knowledge concerning radiation exposure of human populations. Genetic and somatic effects plus effects on growth and development are covered.

235. National Research Council. *The Effects on Populations of Exposure to Low Levels of Ionizing Radiation.* Washington, DC. National Academy of Sciences. 1980.

Familiarly known as BEIR III (Biological Effects of Ionizing Radiation), this is the latest Academy report on effects of low level radiation. Scientific principles in radiation effects as well as sources and rates of exposure are discussed first. Genetic and somatic (cancer and others) effects are then considered. Filled with valuable data. Site specific data is provided for radiation-induced cancers and sites include breast, thyroid, lung, leukemia, esophagus, stomach, etc. Extensively referenced. Glossary. Dissenting reports of committee members regarding the model chosen for risk estimation at low doses are presented.

236. Nenot JC, Stather JW. *The Toxicity of Plutonium, Americium, and Curium.* Oxford. Pergamon Press. 1979.

Prepared under contract for the Commission of the European Communities within its Research and Development Programme on "Plutonium Recycling in Light Water Reactors." Radiological health discussed with respect to the actinides plutonium, americium, and curium. Metabolism and biological effects are stressed in animals and humans. A chapter is devoted to therapy for accidental exposures, especially intravenously administered DTPA for intakes of soluble actinide forms.

237. Olishifski PE, Harford ER, eds. *Industrial Noise and Hearing Conservation*. Chicago. National Safety Council. 1975.

A large and thorough reference text on all aspects of noise and hearing. One chapter of interest classifies various sources of information on noise such as organizations, journals, books, etc. Appendices reprint significant occupational and environmental noise regulations. Glossary.

238. Prasad HN. *Human Radiation Biology*. Hagerstown, MD. Harper and Row. 1974.

A basic textbook about the biological effects of radiation with special attention paid to human tissue. Emphasis on dose-effect relationship. Low level radiation effects included.

239. Sliney D, Wolbarsht M. *Safety with Lasers and Other Optical Sources: A Comprehensive Handbook*. New York. Plenum Press. 1980.

Stresses safety and hazards of lasers but also covers optical exposure from the ambient environment, broad band sources, lighting systems, projection systems, welding arcs, and other optical sources. Concentrates on hazards to the eye and skin, plus safety measures.

240. Upton AC. *Radiation Injury*. Chicago. University of Chicago Press. 1969.

A slim book on the effects of ionizing radiation and its relation to medicine and public health.

241. US Congress. House Committee on Interstate and Foreign Commerce. Subcommittee on Health and the Environment. *Effect of Radiation on Human Health*. Hearings, 95th Congress, 2nd Session. Washington, DC. US Government Printing Office. 1979. [Serial #95-179 and #95-180]

Volume 1, "Health effects of ionizing radiation." Volume 2, "Radiation health effects of medical and diagnostic X-rays."

See also:

De Bruin A. *Biochemical Toxicology of Environmental Agents*. [under *Environmental Toxicology*]

Preger L, ed. *Induced Disease: Drug, Irradiation, Occupation*. [under *Drugs*]

Target Systems

242. Balazs T, ed. *Cardiac Toxicology,* 3 volumes. Boca Raton, FL. CRC Press. 1981.

A broad overview of cardiotoxic agents. Some of the special topics covered are effects on myocardial cells, chemically induced cardiac arrhythmias, coronary no-flow, reversible and irreversible injury. Among the chemicals specifically discussed are inhalation anesthetics, ethanol, digitalis, antihypertensives, antidepressants, antibiotics, fluorocarbons and other industrial chemicals.

243. Chambers PL, Gunzel P. *Mechanisms of Toxic Action on Some Target Organs.* Berlin. Springer-Verlag. 1979.

Supplement 2 of *Archives of Toxicology.* Proceedings of the European Society of Toxicology meeting held in Berlin, June 25-28, 1978. Papers are arranged in sections devoted to the neuro-endocrine system, the liver, and organotropy, plus miscellaneous topics.

244. Davidson CS, Leevy CM, Chamberlayne EC, eds. *Guidelines for Detection of Hepatotoxicity due to Drugs and Chemicals.* Bethesda, MD. US Department of Health, Education and Welfare, Public Health Service, National Institutes of Health. 1979.

(For sale by the Superintendent of Documents, US Government Printing Office, NIH Publication No. 79-313) Represents the combined efforts of internationally recognized authorities. Chapters on histopathology, functional and biochemical evaluation, techniques in detection, drug interactions, preclinical and clinical testing of drugs—all in relation to hepatotoxicity. A concluding chapter considers "sample size considerations for clinical trials of potentially hepatotoxic drugs."

245. Drill VA, Lazar P, eds. *Cutaneous Toxicity.* New York. Academic Press. 1977.

Proceedings of the Third Conference on Cutaneous Toxicity, Washington, DC, May 16-18, 1976. A variety of papers in such areas as cutaneous and percutaneous absorption, surfactants, hair dyes, handwashing, evaluating safety of topical products, and cosmetic legislation.

246. Farber E, Fisher MM, eds. *Toxic Injury of the Liver.* New York. Marcel Dekker. 1979.

A comprehensive compilation of state-of the art reviews on toxic liver injury. Physioanatomical, ultrastructural, biochemical, and immunological bases for toxic liver injury are presented as are the liver's various possible reactions: necrosis, fibrosis, fatty liver, cholestasis. Liver injury by drugs, carcinogens, plant toxins, halogenated hydrocarbons, steroid sex hormones, and alcohol are also discussed.

247. Fisher AA. *Contact Dermatitis,* 2nd ed. Philadelphia. Lea and Febiger. 1973.

Chapters on allergic contact dermatitis, irritant reactions from chemicals, patch testing, effect of metals, clothing, shoes, cosmetics, plants, spices, etc. Includes color photos. An appendix of over 800 contact allergens, their sources of exposure, vehicles for patch testing, and cross reactions.

248. Gilbert HA, Kagan AR, eds. *Radiation Damage to the Nervous System: A Delayed Therapeutic Hazard.* New York. Raven Press. 1980.

Concentrates on brain damage caused by radiation. Additional articles on myelopathy, spinal cord injury, and leukemia.

249. Grant WM. *Toxicology of the Eye,* 2nd ed. Springfield, IL. Charles C. Thomas. 1974.

A major compendium of the effects of drugs, chemicals, plants, and venoms on the eye. Some 1600 substances are covered. Chapter devoted to types of toxic effects influencing vision or the eyes.

250. Lapis K, Johannessen JV. *Liver Carcinogenesis.* Washington, DC. Hemisphere Publishing. 1979.

A state of the art survey of hepatocarcinogenesis as determined from human, animal, and in vitro studies. Covers both viral and chemical carcinogenesis.

251. Manzo L, ed. *Advances in Neurotoxicology.* Oxford. Pergamon Press. 1980.

Proceedings of the International Congress in Neurotoxicology, Varese, Italy, 1979. In 4 sections: metals, alcoholism, occupational and environmental neurotoxins, and drug-induced neurotoxicity. Among the metals discussed are mercury, lead, manganese, and bismuth. Drugs include anticholinergics, antiepileptics, antidepressants, phencyclidine, and lorazepam.

252. Marzulli F, Maibach HI, eds. *Dermatotoxicology and Pharmacology.* Washington, DC. Hemisphere Publishing Corporation. 1977.

Volume 4 of *Advances of Modern Toxicology.* "This volume attempts to provide useful background, reference, and up-to-date state of the art information in areas such as skin irritation, skin sensitization, and skin penetration." Twenty-three chapters in such areas as "Eye Irritation," "Immunological Aspects of Contact Sensitivity," "Intolerance to Food Additives," "Drug and Chemical Induced Hair Loss," and "Cutaneous Carcinogenesis."

253. Mignone L, ed. *Toxic Nephropathies.* Basel. Karger. 1978.

Volume 10 of the series *Contributions to Nephrology* consisting of papers from the 6th International Congress on Toxic Nephropathies held in

Parma in 1977. Papers on nephropathies induced by agents such as gentamicin, D-penicillamine, analgesics, and cadmium.

254. Mokler BV. *Inhalation Toxicology Studies of Aerolized Products.* Albuquerque. Lovelace Biomedical and Environmental Research Institute, Inhalation Toxicology Research Institute. 1979.

(Available from NTIS—PB80-108509) "This report describes an experimental method for assessing the human health risk associated with the use of aerosolized products. The approach was developed and applied to laboratory studies of both cosmetic and household product ingredients."

255. Parkes WR. *Occupational Lung Diseases.* London. Butterworths. 1974.

Diseases caused by dusts, silica, coal and carbon, asbestos, beryllium, and nonmineral organic dusts are within the scope of this monograph. Additional information on the chest radiograph, fate of particles inhaled, particles on the lungs, and even a chapter on basic geology and geochemistry.

256. Simon GA, Paster Z, Klingberg MA, Kaye M, eds. *Skin: Drug Application and Evaluation of Environmental Hazards.* Basel. Karger. 1978.

Volume 7 of *Current Problems in Dermatology.* An excellent overview paper on cutaneous toxicology is followed by papers in such areas as collagen, the scarification test, factors affecting skin permeability, factors affecting percutaneous absorption, lead acetate hair dyes, and housewives' skin and detergents.

257. Smith MB. *Handbook of Ocular Toxicity.* Acton, MA. Publishing Sciences Group. 1976.

Contains brief clinical pharmacology and toxicology data on hazards to the eye of the following groups of substances: abused drugs, nonprescription ocular drugs, other over-the-counter drugs, insecticides, household agents, and assorted commercial chemicals. Appendix of "Ocular Label Warning of Prescription Drugs."

258. Spencer PS, Schaumburg MD, eds. *Experimental and Clinical Neurotoxicology.* Baltimore. Williams and Wilkins. 1980.

A major textbook in the emerging field of neurotoxicology certain to become a standard. In 5 sections: 1. Targets and Classification of Neurotoxic Substances; 2. Pathophysiological Aspects of Toxic-Metabolic Disease; 3. Specific Environmental Neurotoxins; 4. Applied Neurotoxicology; 5. Public Issues and Neurotoxicology. The authors have "tried to encompass the biologist's inquiry into the mechanism of

action of neurotoxic chemicals, the clinical problem of toxic neurological disease, the issues associated with neurotoxicants of environmental
significance, and the regulator's interest in developing sensitive methods
for screening substances for possible neurotoxic effect.'' They have
succeeded admirably.

259. Strik JJTWA, Koeman JH, eds. *Chemical Porphyria in Man.* Amsterdam.
Elsevier/North-Holland Biomedical Press. 1979.

This volume focuses on porphyria in man and experimental animals
induced by halogenated aromatics. Articles on case and experimental
studies, and methods for diagnosis and assessment of chronic hepatic
porphyria.

260. Swanson M, Cook R. *Drugs, Chemicals and Blood Dyscrasias.* Hamilton,
IL. Drug Intelligence Publications. 1977.

Aids health professionals in assessing the likelihood of a particular blood
dyscrasia having been caused by specific drugs or chemicals. The main
portion of this book is an alphabetical list of drugs and chemicals. For
each agent there is information in both prose and tabular form on the
types of abnormalities associated with the substance, the number of
cases reported in the literature, the dose and duration at which the dyscrasia occurred, the mechanism, and references. One index is arranged
alphabetically by blood dyscrasia and permits the user to locate chemicals associated with it. Substances listed range from the ordinary (e.g.,
aspirin, heroin) to the exotic (e.g., Italian beans, moth balls, and wax
crayons).

261. Vinken PJ, Bruyn GW, eds. *Intoxications of the Nervous System.* Amsterdam. North Holland Publishing Company. 1979.

Volumes 36 and 37 of the *Handbook of Clinical Neurology.* These
volumes constitute an excellent encyclopedic compendium of reviews on
various aspects of neurotoxicology. Substances considered for their
neurotoxicity include lead, mercury, arsenic, manganese, thallium, tin,
bromide, phytanic acid, methyl alcohol, solvents, insecticides,
trichloroethylene, mushrooms, snake venoms, marine toxins, antiepilep-
tic drugs, psychotherapeutic agents, hallucinogens, hypnotics, opiates,
salicylate, cardiovascular drugs, and hexachlorophene. Copiously illustrated and referenced.

262. Weiss B, Laties VG, eds. *Behavioral Toxicology.* New York. Plenum
Press. 1975.

Consisting of revisions of papers presented at a 1972 meeting on behavioral toxicology at the University of Rochester. Papers on a variety of

subjects relating to hazards which result in behavioral abnormalities. This is a young and growing branch of toxicology.

263. Zimmerman HJ. *Hepatotoxicity: the Adverse Effects of Drugs and Other Chemicals on the Liver*. New York. Appleton-Century-Crofts. 1978.

A full scale monographic treatment of hepatic injury induced by chemicals. 25 chapters in 4 sections—"General Considerations", "Experimental Hepatotoxicity", "Environmental Hepatotoxicity", and "Iatrogenic Hepatic Injury". Glossaries of drugs and abbreviations. A valuable sourcebook complete with references.

See also:

Environmental Health Perspectives. [under *Periodicals: Specialty Journals–Toxicology*] For conferences on Target Organ Toxicity–Liver and Kidney (v.15), Lung (v.16), Development (v.18), Gonads (v.24), Cardiovascular System, Nervous System (v.26), Intestines (v.33)

Frazier CA. *Occupational Asthma*. [under *Occupational Health and Industrial Hygiene*]

Xintras C. *Behavioral Toxicology*. [under *Occupational Health and Industrial Hygiene*]

Veterinary Toxicology

264. Buck WB, Osweiler GD, Van Gelder GA. *Clinical and Diagnostic Veterinary Toxicology*, 2nd ed. Dubuque, IA. Kendall/Hunt. 1976.

"To present current knowledge on chemical toxicants of significance to livestock production and the welfare of companion animals." Typical headings used throughout chapters include source, toxicity, mechanism of action, clinical signs, physiopathology, diagnosis, and treatment. For toxicologists, instructors, and students of veterinary toxicology, and practicing veterinarians.

265. Clarke EGC, Clarke ML. *Veterinary Toxicology*. London. Bailliere Tindall. 1975.

Primarily a textbook but also a reference work for the practitioner and researcher. Chemicals, poisonous plants, mycotoxins, venomous bites and stings, and radioactive materials are discussed.

266. Keeler RF, van Kampen KR, James LF, eds. *Effects of Poisonous Plants on Livestock*. New York. Academic Press. 1978.

Proceedings of a joint United States-Australian Symposium on Poisonous Plants at Utah State University, Logan, Utah, June 19–24, 1978.

Symposium papers are divided into sections based on the type of toxicity induced—simple phytotoxins, hepatotoxins, cardio/pulmonary toxins, neurotoxins, teratogens and reproductive toxins, and others.

Miscellaneous

267. Albert A. *Selective Toxicity: The Physico-Chemical Basis of Therapy*, 6th ed. London. Chapman and Hall. 1980.

Selectively toxic substances are hazardous to certain cells and not to others. This book basically discusses the mode of action of drugs. Principles of selectivity such as difference in distribution, comparative biochemistry, and comparative cytology are discussed, as are structure-activity relationships.

268. Ballantyne B, ed. *Current Approaches in Toxicology*. Bristol. John Wright and Sons. 1977.

"This volume deals with certain aspects of economic and environmental toxicology. It is the intention to present an overall approach to the requirements for toxicity testing, to draw attention to the various factors influencing the reaction between chemicals and biological materials, to discuss the interpretation of the result of toxicity tests, to describe and critically analyze particular aspects of toxicology of current interest, and to indicate the trends and likely future developments."

269. Boyd EM. *Predictive Toxicometrics: Basic Methods for Estimating Poisonous Amounts of Foods, Drugs, and Other Agents*. Bristol. Scientechnica Publishers. 1972.

"Predictive toxicometrics is the discipline concerned with predicting toxic reactions and the safety of chemical agents in the general population from studies on samples of the same or similar populations." Chapters include "Factorial Toxicometrics," "Uniposal Toxicometrics," and "Multiposal Predictive Toxicometrics." Glossary.

270. Bruce DL. *Functional Toxicity of Anesthesia*. New York. Grune and Stratton. 1980.

One book in the series, *The Scientific Basis of Clinical Anesthesia*. "Were there no ill effects attendant to anesthetics, there would be no need for experts to administer them. Since there *are* such effects, anesthesiologists must learn to anticipate, treat, and most of all, avoid them whenever possible. The purpose of this monograph has been to aid these individuals in achieving those goals." Divided into functions of central nervous system, circulation, respiration, kidney, liver, endocrine system, and cell division.

271. Cohen Y, ed. *Toxicology*. Oxford. Pergamon Press. 1979.

Volume 9 in *Advances in Pharmacology and Therapeutics*. Proceedings of the 7th International Congress of Pharmacology, Paris, 1978. A broad range of articles in the areas of reactive metabolites, behavioral toxicology, and topical applications.

272. Fawcett DW, Newberne JW, eds. *Workshop on Cellular and Molecular Toxicology*. Baltimore. Williams and Wilkins. 1980.

Workshop convened by the Pharmaceutical Manufacturers Association. Investigated toxic effects at the cellular and molecular level. Sessions on the cell surface, cytoplasmic membrane systems, the cell nucleus, mutagenesis, and lysosomes. A concluding chapter by Gerhard Zbinden entitled "Application of Basic Concepts of Research to Toxicology."

273. Filov VA, Golubev AA, Liublina EI, Tolokontsvev NA. *Quantitative Toxicology: Selected Topics*. New York. John Wiley. 1979.

This is an English language revised and enlarged edition of the 1973 Russian book, *Kolichestvennaya Toksikologiya*. The translation is by VE Tatarchenko. A highly mathematical account of toxicology. Some of the topics featured are "The Equilibrium Distribution of Nonelectrolytes between the Environment and the Living Organism," "Kinetic Aspects of the Absorption and Fate of Poisons in the Body," "Methods for the Calculation of Toxicity Parameters and Maximum Allowable Concentrations."

274. Galli CL, Murphy SD, Paoletti R, eds. *The Principles and Methods in Modern Toxicology*. Amsterdam. Elsevier/North-Holland. 1980.

Proceedings of the International Course on the Principles and Methods of Modern Toxicology held in Belgirate, Italy in 1979. This is volume 6 of the *Symposia of the Giovanni Lorenzini Foundation*. A general monograph on a miscellany of topics such as toxicity testing, reproductive toxicity, toxicologic pathology, choice of animal species, immunity, and good laboratory practice.

275. Hunter WJ, Smeets JGPM, eds. *The Evaluation of Toxicological Data for the Protection of Human Health*. Oxford. Pergamon Press. 1977.

Based on a 1976 International Colloquium held in Luxembourg and organized by the Commission of the European Communities and the International Academy of Environmental Safety. Provides critical reviews of toxicological tests, evaluation of data and concepts of safe levels. Also covers ecotoxicological approaches for the protection of health and the environment.

276. Jakoby WB, ed. *Enzymatic Basis of Detoxication,* 2 volumes. New York. Academic Press. 1980.

These are the first 2 volumes of a series of monographs entitled *Biochemical Pharmacology and Toxicology.* They present "the current state of our knowledge of foreign compound metabolism at the level of what specific enzymes can do." Among the broad topics covered are physiological aspects, mixed function oxygenase systems and other oxidation-reduction systems (e.g. alcohol dehydrogenase, aldehyde reductase), conjugation reactions, and hydrolytic systems.

277. Jollow DJ, Kocsis JJ, Snyder R, Vainio H, eds. *Biological Reactive Intermediates: Formation, Toxicity, and Inactivation.* New York. Plenum Press. 1977.

Proceedings of an International Conference on Active Intermediates held at the University of Turku, Turku, Finland, July 26–27, 1975. Covalent binding, formation, and inactivation of reactive intermediates, and their roles in lipid peroxidation and carcinogenesis are topics covered. Some of the specific chemicals discussed are hydrazines, nitrite, benzene, carbon disulfide, benzo(a)pyrene, diazepam, and paracetamol. The key points of the conference discussions are summarized.

278. Kaiser HE. *Species-Specific Potential of Invertebrates for Toxicological Research.* Baltimore. University Park Press. 1980.

"This state of the art review is intended to induce interested scientists, especially those working in the fields of experimental pathology and experimental toxicology to a more advanced use of invertebrates as animal models. It is the first attempt to treat all invertebrate phyla in one book compilation under the aspects of intoxification, disease, or abnormal function." References on five microfiche cards.

279. *Kirk-Othmer Encyclopedia of Chemical Technology,* 3rd ed. New York. John Wiley. 1978–1984(?).

Undoubtedly the finest scientific encyclopedia available, covering much more than its title would suggest. The third edition, being published in stages, is scheduled for completion (24 volumes plus an index) in 1984. The first 11 volumes were available by the end of 1980. An excellent source for information on the toxicology of products or processes and much more supporting information. Chemical abstracts registry numbers are used throughout. Authors and their affiliations are identified for all entries.

280. Lowrance WW. *Of Acceptable Risk: Science and the Determination of Safety.* Los Altos, CA. William Kaufmann. 1976.

Of particular interest to those involved in or concerned with the legislative process and the rationale behind decision-making. A cogent analysis of the measurement of risk and the judgement of safety. Stimulating material for anyone interested in societal and ethical issues in toxicology.

281. Mehlman MA, Shapiro RE, Cranmer MF, Norvell MJ, eds. *Hazards from Toxic Chemicals*. Park Forest, IL, Pathotox Publishers. 1978.

Proceedings of the Second Annual Conference on the Status of Predictive Tools in Application to Safety Evaluation. Cosponsored by the National Center for Toxicological Research and the National Institutes of Health. Proceedings devoted mostly to carcinogens, subcellular toxicological evaluation, information technology in prediction of toxic hazards, and teratological testing.

282. Mehlman MA, Shapiro RE, Blumenthal H, eds. *New Concepts in Safety Evaluation*. Washington, DC. Hemisphere Publishing. Part 1, 1976; Part 2, 1979.

Volume 1 of *Advances in Modern Toxicology*. In Part 1, conceptual and methodological tools, pharmacokinetics, metabolism, and food and environmental interactions are all discussed in relation to evaluating the safety of foreign compounds. One chapter is devoted to safety evaluation with regard to diethylstilbestrol. Part 2 treats environmental carcinogenesis (including epidemiology, extrapolation, and risk estimation), metal-tissue interactions, biomaterials, nitrosamines, illicit drugs, and target organ studies.

283. Miller MW and Shamoo AE, eds. *Membrane Toxicity*. New York. Plenum Press. 1977.

This, the proceedings of the 9th Rochester International Conference on Environmental Toxicity, is volume 84 of *Advances in Experimental Medicine and Biology*. The book evaluates "present concepts of membrane structure and function in relation to exposure to environmental toxicants."

284. National Fire Protection Association. *Fire Protection Guide on Hazardous Materials*. 7th ed. Boston. National Fire Protection Association. 1978.

285. Paget GE, ed. *Good Laboratory Practice*. Baltimore. University Park Press. 1979.

Part of the *Topics in Toxicology* series sponsored by Inveresk Research International. Adequate standards for toxicity testing are discussed. Regulatory aspects in the US, Italy, and Great Britain, data audits, GLP in a pathology lab, the viewpoint of the animal breeder, and hardware solutions are among the topics discussed in relation to GLP.

285a. Paget GE, Thomson R, eds. *Standard Operating Procedures in Toxicology.* Lancaster, England. MTP Press. 1979.

Developed by Edinburgh's Inveresk Research International Limited, this publication consists of their Code of Good Laboratory Practice and Standard Operating Procedures. Procedures for record keeping, test substances, and general toxicology. Specific documentation for non-species specific, mice, rats, rabbits, dogs, and primates. Contains sample forms.

286. Plaa GL, Duncan WAM, eds. *Proceedings of the First International Congress on Toxicology: Toxicology as a Predictive Science.* New York. Academic Press. 1978.

This congress, initiated by the European Society of Toxicology and the Society of Toxicology, "covered all fields of toxicology and emphasis was given to reports that would encourage the formulation of hypotheses and toxicological research so that the prediction of potential toxicological hazards would be improved".

287. Stockholm International Peace Research Institute. *Medical Protection against Chemical-Warfare Agents.* Stockholm. Almqvist and Wiksell. 1976.

The chemical-warfare agents under consideration are primarily organophosphorous nerve agents. Atropine and oxime therapy are among the treatments discussed.

288. Toxic Substance Strategy Committee. *Toxic Chemicals and Public Protection: A Report to the President by the Toxic Substances Strategy Committee.* Washington, DC. Council on Environmental Quality. 1980.

Reviews the work of the Toxic Substance Strategy committee and presents its conclusions and recommendations concerning the health risks of toxic chemicals. Topics discussed are chemical information systems, confidentiality, research in support of regulation, response to crises, regulatory programs, and carcinogens. In addition, a chapter is devoted to the international scene and outlines significant organizations, problems, and policies.

289. World Health Organization. *Methods Used in the USSR for Establishing Biologically Safe Levels of Toxic Substances.* Geneva. World Health Organization. 1975.

Consisting of papers presented at a WHO meeting in Moscow, 1972. A succinct, if somewhat sketchy and perhaps outdated, assessment of criteria for toxicity testing and standard setting in the Soviet Union. Russian toxicologists believe that ''in all countries... hygienic standards should have the force of law and should not be mere recommendations.'' Useful for comparison and contrast with US methods.

Chapter 3

Special Monographs

Three of the four following monographic series are produced by specialist panels selected for their expertise in certain areas of toxicology. The *IARC Scientific Publications* series, although not committee produced, have been placed in this section because of their strong ties to the *IARC Monographs*. The objective of the latter program has been stated by IARC as being "... to elaborate and publish in the form of monographs critical reviews of data on carcinogenicity for groups of chemicals to which humans are known to be exposed, to evaluate these data in terms of human risk with the help of international working groups of experts in chemical carcinogenesis and related fields, and to indicate where additional research efforts are needed." An enormous amount of effort and expense is involved in the production of these high-quality critical reviews and syntheses of the carcinogenicity literature. Single issues of both of the aforementioned IARC publications are available from the WHO Publications Centre USA, 49 Sheridan Avenue, Albany, NY 12210 or the Franklin Institute Press, Benjamin Franklin Parkway, Philadelphia, PA 19103. Subscription information may be obtained from the World Health Organization, Distribution and Sales, 1211 Geneva 27, Switzerland.

The *Medical and Biologic Effects of Environmental Pollutants* series prepared by various expert subcommittees of the Committee on Medical and Biologic Effects of Environmental Pollutants, Division of Medical Sciences, Assembly of Life Sciences, National Research Council, provides in-depth, extensively referenced analyses of chemicals or classes of chemicals which are potential or known hazards to man or to which there is wide exposure. The volumes in this series were originally published by the National Academy of Sciences in Washington, DC. More recent volumes have been published by University Park Press in Baltimore. The National Academy of Sciences is still publishing reports prepared by expert committees, such as the one on lead (see chapter 2: Books, Metals), though these are no longer with the Committee on Medical and Biological Effects. *Environmental Health Criteria* is published under the joint sponsorship of the United Nations Environment Programme and the World Health Organization. The documents concentrate on factors and agents that may adversely affect man. They must have relevance to human health.

IARC Monographs on the Evaluation of the Carcinogenic Risk of Chemicals to Humans

IARC Monographs on the Evaluation of the Carcinogenic Risk of Chemicals to Humans

Lyon. International Agency for Research on Cancer. 17, 1978– [Continues *IARC Monographs on the Evaluation of the Carcinogenic Risk of Chemicals to Man*]

290. *Some Inorganic Substances, Chlorinated Hydrocarbons, Aromatic Amines, N-Nitroso Compounds, and Natural Products.* 1, 1972.

291. *Some Inorganic and Organometallic Compounds.* 2, 1973.

292. *Certain Polycyclic Aromatic Hydrocarbons and Heterocyclic Compounds.* 3, 1973.

293. *Some Aromatic Amines, Hydrazine and Related Substances, N-Nitroso Compounds and Miscellaneous Alkylating Agents.* 4, 1974.

294. *Some Organochlorine Pesticides.* 5, 1974.

295. *Sex Hormones.* 6, 1974.

296. *Some Anti-Thyroid and Related Substances, Nitrofurans and Related Substances, Nitrofurans and Industrial Chemicals.* 7, 1974.

297. *Some Aromatic Azo Compounds.* 8, 1975.

298. *Some Aziridines, N-, S-, and O-Mustards and Selenium.* 9, 1975.

299. *Some Naturally Occurring Substances.* 10, 1976.

300. *Cadmium, Nickel, Some Epoxides, Miscellaneous Industrial Chemicals and General Considerations on Volatile Anaesthetics.* 11, 1976.

301. *Some Carbamates, Thiocarbamates and Carbazides.* 12, 1976.

302. *Some Miscellaneous Pharmaceutical Substances.* 13, 1977.

303. *Asbestos.* 14, 1977.

304. *Some Fumigants, the Herbicides 2,4-D and 2,4,5-T, Chlorinated Dibenzodioxins and Miscellaneous Industrial Chemicals.* 15, 1977.

305. *Some Aromatic Amines and Related Nitro Compounds—Hair Dyes, Colouring Agents and Miscellaneous Industrial Chemicals.* 16, 1978.

306. *Some N-Nitroso Compounds.* 17, 1978.

307. *Polychlorinated Biphenyls and Polybrominated Biphenyls.* 18, 1978.

308. *Some Monomers, Plastics and Synthetic Elastomers and Acrolein.* 19, 1979.

309. *Some Halogenated Hydrocarbons.* 20, 1979.

310. *Chemicals and Industrial Processes Associated with Cancer in Humans.* Supplement 1, 1979.

311. *Sex Hormones (II).* 21, 1979.

312. *Some Non-Nutritive Sweetening Agents.* 22, 1980.

312a. *Some Pharmaceutical Drugs.* 24, 1980.

313. *Some Metals and Metallic Compounds.* 23, 1980.

314. *Long Term and Short Term Screening Assays for Carcinogens: A Critical Appraisal.* Supplement 2, 1980.

IARC Scientific Publications

Lyon. International Agency for Research on Cancer. 1, 1971–

315. *Liver Cancer.* 1, 1971.

316. *Onconogenesis and Herpesviruses.* 2, 1972.

317. *N-Nitroso Compounds Analysis and Formation.* 3, 1972.

318. *Transplacental Carcinogenesis.* 4, 1973.

319. *Pathology of Tumours in Laboratory Animals. Volume I. Tumours of the Rat. Part I.* 5, 1973.

320. *Pathology of Tumours in Laboratory Animals. Volume I. Tumours of the Rat. Part II.* 6, 1973.

321. *Host Environment Interactions in the Etiology of Cancer in Man.* 7, 1973.

322. *Biological Effects of Asbestos.* 8, 1973.

323. *N-Nitroso Compounds in the Environment.* 9, 1974.

324. *Chemical Carcinogenesis Essays.* 10, 1974.

325. *Oncogenesis and Herpesviruses.* 11, 1975.

326. *Screening Tests in Chemical Carcinogenesis.* 12, 1976.

327. *Environmental Pollution and Carcinogenic Risks.* 13, 1976.

328. *Environmental N-Nitroso Compounds-Analysis and Formation.* 14, 1976.

329. *Cancer Incidence in Five Continents—Volume III.* 15, 1976.

330. *Air Pollution and Cancer in Man.* 16, 1977.

331. *Directory of On-Going Research in Cancer Epidemiology.* 17, 1977.

332. *Environmental Carcinogens-Selected Methods of Analysis. Volume I: Analysis of Volatile Nitrosamines in Food.* 18, 1978.

333. *Environmental Aspects of N-Nitroso Compounds.* 19, 1978.

334. *Nasopharyngeal Carcinoma: Etiology and Control.* 20, 1978.

335. *Cancer Registration and its Techniques.* 21, 1978.

336. *Environmental Carcinogens-Selected Methods of Analysis. Volume II: Vinyl Chloride.* 22, 1978.

337. *Pathology of Tumours in Laboratory Animals. Volume II. Tumours of the Mouse.* 23, 1979.

338. *Oncogenesis and Herpesviruses III.* 24, 1978.

339. *Carcinogenic Risks: Strategies for Intervention.* 25, 1979.

340. *Directory of On-Going Research in Cancer Epidemiology 1978.* 26, 1978.

341. *Molecular and Cellular Aspects of Carcinogen Screening Tests.* 27, 1980.

342. *Directory of On-Going Research in Cancer Epidemiology 1979.* 28, 1979.

343. *Environmental Carcinogens-Selected Methods of Analysis. Volume III: Polycyclic Aromatic Hydrocarbons.* 29, 1979.

344. *Handling Chemical Carcinogens in the Laboratory: Problems of Safety.* 33, 1979.

345. *Directory of On-Going Research in Cancer Epidemiology 1980.* 35, 1980.

National Research Council: Medical and Biological Effects of Environmental Pollutants

National Research Council. Committee on Medical and Biological Effects of Environmental Pollutants. *Medical and Biological Effects of Environmental Pollutants.* Published variously by the National Academy of Sciences, Washington DC, and University Park Press, Baltimore.

346. *Airborne Particles.* 1979.

> "The emphasis of this report . . . is on particles that result from man's activities. The types of particles and their distribution are considered. The origins, behavior and fate of such particles, their physical and chemical interactions . . . monitoring . . . deposition, clearance, and retention of particles, and their effects on man and on other animals . . . epidemiologic evidence . . . effects of particulate matter on vegetation and materials."

347. *Ammonia.* 1979.

> Effects on both man and materials are covered as are properties, monitoring, sources, and toxicology. The Ammonia Subcommittee calls for increased research efforts in understanding hepatic coma, high tolerance of

bats to atmospheric ammonia, pulmonary effects in animals, late sequelae of acute inhalation and chronic exposure, etc. Extensive list of references.

348. *Arsenic.* 1977.

Chemistry, distribution, metabolism, toxicity in plants, animals, man. Appendices on arsenic content of plants and animals. Glossary. Subcommittee on Arsenic recommends further studies on arsenic toxicity, especially on the role of arsenic in carcinogenicity. The Subcommittee also recommends that the use of the rat be discouraged in experiments on arsenic metabolism because this animal's arsenic metabolism varies so widely from man or other mammals.

349. *Chlorine and Hydrogen Chloride.* 1976.

Health and other effects of chlorine and hydrogen chloride. Chapter on the safe handling of these chemicals.

350. *Copper.* 1977.

Focuses on copper and copper metabolism in plants, animals, and man, and occupational and community exposures to the element. Includes a glossary of compounds and an appendix on "Copper analysis in environmental and biologic samples."

351. *Fluorides.* 1971.

The Panel on Flourides recommends increased industrial studies of groups exposed to airborne flourides. This monograph also evaluated hazards of various populations exposed to fluorides in the air or water supply.

352. *Hydrogen Sulfide.* 1979.

Effects on man, animals, vegetation, and aquatic life. One chapter devoted to "The physiological and aesthetic aspects of odor". A high priority recommendation by the Subcommittee that prepared this report is for future research on the effects of long term low level exposures.

353. *Iron.* 1979.

Discusses iron metabolism, deficiency, acute and chronic toxicities, and iron inhalation.

354. *Lead: Airborne Lead in Perspective.* 1972.

Airborne lead and lead alkyl compounds are studied—their biological effects in man as well as on domestic and wild animals.

355. *Manganese.* 1973.

Discusses biochemistry and metabolism of manganese as well as epidemiology of manganese intoxication, permissible air concentrations, and neurobehavioral effects.

356. *Nickel.* 1975.

Special areas of nickel toxicity examined are nickel and dermal responses, nickel carcinogenesis, and nickel and the reproductive system. An appendix provides ambient nickel concentrations as reported by air surveillance networks throughout the country.

357. *Nitrogen Oxides.* 1977.

As a primary product of fossil fuel combustion, nitrogen oxides are likely to be with us for some time. Effects of these compounds are considered on ecosystems, materials, vegetation, man and animals. The Nitrogen Oxides Subcommittee recommends increased research on human lung function, on the relationship between animal respiratory infections and nitrogen dioxide, and on the relationship between long-term exposures and chronic respiratory disease.

358. *Ozone and Other Photochemical Oxidants.* 1977.

A detailed description of photochemical oxidants and their effects on the environment and biological systems. Epidemiologic and controlled studies on humans are discussed as is respiratory transport, ecosystems, toxicology, and effects on plants and microorganisms. Includes recommendations for future research.

359. *Platinum-Group Metals.* 1977.

Sources, properties, uses, analysis, toxicology and pharmacology. Chapter on allergic response to platinum compounds.

360. *Polycyclic Organic Matter.* 1972.

The emphasis in this monograph is on aspects of carcinogenesis, such as testing, experimental design, in-vivo and in-vitro approaches. Other topics are teratogenesis, mutagenesis, and clinical and epidemiologic studies.

361. *Selenium.* 1976.

362. *Vanadium.* 1974.

Covers industrial processes involving uses of vanadium. The many industrial and community exposures to vanadium are discussed. Appendices on "Desulfurization of residual fuel oils" and "Detection and measurement of vanadium in biologic and pollution materials."

363. *Vapor-phase organic pollutants.* 1976.

363a. *Zinc.* 1979.

Properties and sources of zinc. Zinc in plants, aquatic organisms, man, the diet, metalloproteins. Clinical aspects, toxicity, environmental standards and sampling techniques. Appendices on content of zinc in foods and zinc analysis. 1855 references.

Environmental Health Criteria

364. *Environmental Health Criteria.* Geneva. World Health Organization. 1, 1976–

Mercury. 1, 1976.

Polychlorinated Biphenyls and Terphenyls. 2, 1976.

Lead. 3, 1977.

Oxides of Nitrogen. 4, 1977.

Nitrates, Nitrites, and N-Nitroso Compounds. 5, 1977.

Principles and Methods for Evaluating the Toxicity of Chemicals, Part 1. 6, 1978.

Photochemical Oxidants. 7, 1978.

Sulfur Oxides and Suspended Particulate Matter. 8, 1979.

DDT and its Derivatives. 9, 1979.

Carbon Disulfide. 10, 1979.

Mycotoxins. 11, 1979.

Noise. 12, 1980.

Carbon Monoxide. 13, 1979.

Ultraviolet Radiation. 14, 1979.

Tin and Organotin Compounds. 15, 1980.

Chapter 4

Annual Reports

Virtually all the organizations listed in this book issue annual reports and these are always good publications to consult for information regarding the agency's activities. This section lists a small number of annual reports which may be particularly useful as reference tools and which describe ventures outside of those in which the issuing agency, itself, may be engaged. The citations are to the latest issues to which I had access. For current information, the reader should request the most recent annual report from the agency. The annotations refer to the particular issues cited and do not necessarily reflect the content of past or future reports.

365. *Council on Environmental Quality*

> *Environmental Quality—1980: The eleventh annual report of the Council on Environmental Quality.* [available from GPO - stock no. 041-011-00047-5]

A very informative monograph outlining the state of the environment. Chapters on air, water, toxic substances, municipal solid wastes, energy, natural resources, ecology, noise, the National Environmental Policy Act, the global environment, and economics. Includes excellent tables, figures, charts, and graphs containing useful environmental data. One of the best books to consult on recent issues and events relating to the environment and toxicology.

366. *National Institute of Environmental Health Sciences*

> Schambra PE. *Federal agency support for environmental health research: A report by the National Institute of Environmental Health*

Sciences. Research Triangle Park, North Carolina, National Institute of Environmental Health Sciences, 1980.

This annual report provides an overview of environmental health research activities and funding. Detailed descriptions are given for programs of agencies with environmental health research responsibilities. A valuable appendix lists interagency coordinative groups broken down into areas such as "General Coordinating Groups," "Specialized Coordinating Groups," "Special Populations Coordinating Groups," "Toxic Substances/Effluents Coordinating Groups," "Carcinogenesis/Mutagenesis/Reproductive/Metabolic Effects Coordinating Groups", "Energy Effects Coordinating Groups," "Oceanic/Atmospheric/Climatic Coordinating Groups," "Ionizing Radiation Coordinating Groups," etc. This annual report can serve as a directory of federal groups doing environmental health-related research.

367. *National Toxicology Program*

Review of current DHEW research related to toxicology and Annual Report. National Toxicology Program, Public Health Service, Department of Health, Education and Welfare. 1980. [available from National Institute of Environmental Health Sciences. P.O. Box 12233. Research Triangle Park, NC—#NTP-79-7]

Extremely useful tools outlining DHEW activities in toxicology research. In the "Review of Research," the NTP asks each agency for information on basic toxicology research, toxicology testing, and toxicology method development. A table outlines funding expected in each of these areas. Listed are descriptions of research in textual and tabular form. Specific chemicals being tested are named, along with type of test being performed, etc. The "Annual Plan" provides a basic overview of the plan plus information on organization, toxicology research and testing activities, and coordinative management activities.

Chapter 5

Fugitive Literature

"Fugitive Literature" is the rather imprecise term I have chosen to define items of a somewhat elusive nature, those that are generally more difficult to locate and acquire than traditional books and periodicals. Many of these are reports coming out of associations and government agencies. Often documents on regulations or policy are published in the *Federal Register*. Some of the publications are skimpy and ephemeral. Others, such as the *Survey of Compounds* and the *TSCA Inventory* are enormous undertakings of lasting reference value. This is a very brief selection of both the very well known (e.g., *NIOSH Criteria Documents*) and the more obscure (e.g., *CIIT Current Status Reports*). It is almost impossible to keep up with all of this publicly available documentation. Probably the best approach is to select as many organizations as there are relevant to your specific job, make contacts within them if possible, and get your name on mailing lists.

Both *Government Reports Announcements* and the *Monthly Catalogue of United States Government Publications* (see *Abstracts, Indexes and Current Awareness*) may be consulted for the less obscure fugitive literature.

368. *Calendar of Federal Regulations*
Washington, DC. United States Regulatory Council.

Published in May and November of each year as a special issue of the *Federal Register,* this calendar catalogs significant Federal regulations under development. Arranged by agency. For each proposed standard or regulation, information such as the following is listed: the legal authority for the standard or regulation, a statement of the problem, alternatives under consideration, summaries of benefits and costs, sectors affected, related regulations and actions, government collaboration, a timetable (for notice of proposed rulemaking, public hearing, final rule, etc.), available documents pertaining to the rulemaking, and an agency contact person (with address and phone number).

369. *CIIT Current Status Reports*
Research Triangle Park, NC. Chemical Industry Institute of Toxicology.

Reports on toxic effects of chemicals. Chemicals already done include n-hexane and dinitrotoluene.

370. *Chemical Hazard Information Profiles (CHIPS): August 1976–August 1978*
Washington, DC. Environmental Protection Agency. Office of Pesticides and Toxic Substances. 1980.

Part of EPA's *TSCA Chemical Assessment Series.* Brief profiles of 43 chemicals chosen "on the basis of information indicating a potential for adverse health or environmental effects, along with evidence of commercial production or environmental exposure." Preparation of these profiles is the Office of Pesticides and Toxic Chemicals' first step in the assessment of chemicals.

370a. *CHRIS (Chemical Hazard Response Information System).*
Washington, DC. Department of Transportation. US Coast Guard.

CHRIS "is designed to provide information needed for decisionmaking by responsible Coast Guard personnel during emergencies that occur during the water transport of hazardous chemicals". The components of *CHRIS* include *A condensed guide to chemical hazards, Hazardous chemical data, Hazard assessment handbook, Response methods handbook,* and the *Hazard assessment computer system. The Hazardous Chemical Data* manual is considered the major component of the system. Among the data provided for each chemical is labelling, response to discharge, nomenclature, physical and chemical properties, health hazards (including toxicity data), fire hazards, chemical reactivity, water pollution, manufacturers and shipping information.

371. *Cosmetic Ingredient Review Summary of Scientific Literature on . . .*
Washington, DC. Cosmetic Ingredient Review.

Summaries of information obtained from the open literature on cosmetics and cosmetic ingredients.

372. *Department of Labor, Occupational Safety and Health Administration. Identification, Classification and Regulation of Potential Occupational Carcinogens.* In *The Federal Register,* Tuesday, Jan. 22, 1980, Book 2 of 2 Books.

Also known as the OSHA Cancer Policy, this document "provides for future individual rulemakings concerning each substance, or combination or mixture of substances, or process to be regulated, thereby affording the public and OSHA the opportunity, among other things, to determine the applicability of this general policy to any specific substance, combination or mixture of substances or process and to select the most effective type of regulation to control human exposures to such potential occupational carcinogenic substance, combination or mixture of substances or process.''

373. *EPA Chemical Activities Status Report*
Washington, DC. Environmental Protection Agency. Office of Pesticides and Toxic Substances. 1979.

Part of the *Toxics Integration Information Series*. ''. . . organizes data on EPA's many programs to assess and regulate chemical substances and mixtures. It catalogues both the completed and on-going work of the Office of Toxic Substances and other EPA program offices. These data will alert those beginning assessment and control activities—including surveys, investigations, monitoring, and rule development—to related programs completed or underway in EPA.''

374. *First Annual Report on Carcinogens*
Department of Health and Human Services, National Toxicology Program. 1980.

Brings together in one source the data collected by various agencies on carcinogens and their regulation. The report is based heavily on the 26 chemicals or industrial processes identified by the IARC Monograph series as being strongly associated with human cancers.

375. *Identification, Classification and Regulation of Potential Occupational Carcinogens*
In the *Federal Register* 45(15), Book 2 of 2, Jan 22 1980.

Better known as OSHA's ''Cancer Policy'', this final rule is OSHA's policy for substances posing potential occupational carcinogenic risk to humans.

376. *Interagency Regulatory Liaison Group Regulatory Reporter*
Washington, DC. Sigma Dat Computing Corp.

This publication prepared for the IRLG under contract to CEQ outlines the IRLG's integrative and coordinating activities of their various chemical task groups. Background information on the chemicals, a schedule of actions taken, current status of the chemical and current agency technical contacts with phone numbers are provided.

377. *National Cancer Institute Carcinogenesis Technical Report Series*
Bethesda, MD: National Institutes of Health.

In-depth reports on the results of bioassays of chemicals selected for the Carcinogenesis Testing Program. Contains occasional guidelines for animal bioassay.

378. *NIOSH Criteria for a Recommended Standard . . .*
National Institute for Occupational Safety and Health.

NIOSH evaluates all available research data and criteria for chemicals or classes of chemicals and recommends standards for occupational exposure. Among the dozens of substances for which criteria documents have been prepared are acetylene, acrylamide, acrylonitrile, alkanes, allyl chloride, ammonia, antimony, asbestos, asphalt fumes, benzene, waste anesthetic gases and vapors, xylene, and zinc oxide. See also the massive *NIOSH Publications Catalog,* 4th ed. Cincinnati. NIOSH Division of Technical Services. 1980. (DHHS (NIOSH) Publication No. 80-126) which lists and provides ordering information for all NIOSH documents including the Criteria Documents.

379. *NTP Technical Bulletin*
Department of Health and Human Services, National Toxicology Program. 1, 1980–

Details on the status of chemicals and other activities within NTP.

380. *SCOGS Reports*
Bethesda, MD. Federation of American Societies for Experimental Biology.

A series investigating the use of GRAS (Generally Recognized as Safe) food substances or ingredients.

381. *Survey of Compounds which have been tested for Carcinogenic Activity*
Bethesda, MD. National Cancer Institute. 1941–

Prepared for the National Cancer Institute by the Franklin Research Center. The fifth and most recent volume of this massive undertaking was published in 1978 and contains only documents published in 1978. ''The survey consists entirely of carcinogenesis data extracted from published information and arranged in a uniform tabular format.'' The tables are highly structured and allow for easy access to data and findings of experiments. Categories for each article include the animal studied, strain, sex, preparation and dose of substance administered, route and site, number of animals with various specified tumors, survival rates, and the duration of the experiment.

382. *Toxic Substance Control Act: Initial Inventory*
Washington, DC. United States Environmental Protection Agency. 1979.

Six volume inventory of all chemical substances in the US not regulated by other agencies. 44,000 chemicals are in the initial inventory. The cumulative supplement published on July 30, 1980 brings the total Revised Inventory up to 55,103 chemical substances. Manufacturers who do not have their chemicals in the inventory are required to go through pre-manufacturing notification as stipulated in TOSCA.

383. *TLV's: Threshold Limit Values for Chemical Substances and Physical Agents in the Workroom Environment with Intended Changes for . . .*
Cincinnati, OH. American Conference of Governmental Industrial Hygienists.

ACGIH has tried to set TLV's for chemical substances and physical agents which represent the limit below which workers may be daily exposed without adverse effect. This handbook is published annually.

384. *TSCA Chemical Assessment Series*
Washington, DC. United States Environmental Protection Agency, Office of Pesticides and Toxic Substances.

Chemical evaluations issued as part of TSCA implementation.

385. *TSCA Chemicals-in-Progress Bulletin*
Washington, DC. United States Environmental Protection Agency, Office of Pesticides and Toxic Substances. 1, 1980–

A news bulletin outlining developments concerning the Toxic Substances Control Act.

Chapter 6

Popular Works

The distinction between popular and technical works is somewhat arbitrary. Popular articles and editorials may appear in otherwise technical journals. Generally, popular works are written at a level requiring minimal subject expertise and are addressed to a lay audience. The better popular works provide quite interesting and informative reading and may even be a good starting point for a scientific investigator seeking a social perspective.

There are many sources available for locating popular works and current event literature. Among these are: public libraries, *Books in Print* (a,b) and its subject guide, *The Readers' Guide* (c), *PAIS* (d), *The New York Times Index* (c), and data bases to general periodical literature.

Popular articles on toxicology have appeared in such unlikely sources as *Glamour Magazine, McCalls,* and *Rolling Stone.* The subject pervades newspapers and other news media. More likely than not, each day's edition of major city newspapers will report on an oil spill, a radiation accident, chemicals determined to be carcinogenic, drug effects, pesticide poisonings, birth defects, occupational diseases, air pollution, cosmetic recalls, etc.

Many popular books and investigative journalism, despite occasionally questionable scientific validity, have been influential in bringing serious problems to light and have sparked increased research. *Silent Spring,* for instance, was extremely important in the growth of the environmental movement.

References

(a) *Books in Print*. New York. Bowker.

(b) *Subject Guide to Books in Print*. New York. Bowker.

(c) *Public Affairs Information Service Bulletin* New York. Public Affairs Information Service. 1, 1915–

(d) *Readers' Guide to Periodical Literature*. New York. H. W. Wilson. 1900–

(e) *The New York Times Index*. New York. The New York Times. 1, 1851–

386. Brown M. *Laying Waste: The Poisoning of America by Toxic Chemicals*. New York. Pantheon Press. 1980.

387. Carson R. *Silent Spring*. Boston. Houghton Mifflin. 1962.

388. Corbett TH. *Cancer and Chemicals*. Chicago. Nelson-Hall. 1977.

389. Environmental Defense Fund. *Malignant Neglect*. New York. Random House. 1980.

390. Feingold BF. *Why Your Child is Hyperactive*. New York. Random House. 1975.

391. Fuller JG. *200,000,000 Guinea Pigs; New Dangers in Everyday Foods, Drugs and Cosmetics*. East Rutherford, NJ. Putnam. 1972.

392. Gofman JW, Tamplin AR. *Poisoned Power: Case against Nuclear Power Plants*. Emmaus, PA. Rodale Press. 1971.

393. Griffiths J, Ballantine R. *Silent Slaughter*. Chicago. Regnery. 1972.

394. Hardin JW, Arena JM. *Human Poisoning from Native and Cultivated Plants*. Durham, NC. Duke University Press. 1974.

395. Hunter BT. *Food Additives and Federal Policy: The Mirage of Safety*. New York. Charles Scribner's Sons. 1975.

396. Lipscomb DM. *Noise: The Unwanted Sounds*. Chicago. Nelson-Hall. 1974.

397. Lucas J. *Our Polluted Food: A Survey of the Risks*. New York. John Wiley. 1974.

398. Norwood C. *At Highest Risk: Environmental Hazards to Young and Un-born Children*. New York. McGraw-Hill. 1979.

399. Schroeder HA. *The Poisons around Us: Toxic Metals in Food, Air, and Water*. Bloomington. Indiana University Press. 1974.

400. Verrett J. *Eating May Be Hazardous to Your Health*. New York. Simon and Schuster. 1974.

401. Wellford H. *Sowing the Wind*. New York. Grossman Publishers. 1972.

402. Wertheim AH. *The Natural Poisons in Natural Foods*. Secucus, NJ. Stuart. 1974.

403. Whelan EM. *Preventing Cancer*. New York. Norton. 1978.

404. Whiteside.T *The Pendulum and the Toxic Cloud: the Course of Dioxin Contamination*. New Haven. Yale University Press. 1979.

405. Winter R. *Cancer Causing Agents: A Preventive Guide*. New York. Crown. 1979.

Chapter 7

Periodicals

The list of specialty journals in toxicology are professional journals which devote the bulk of their space to articles highly relevant to toxicology. The brief list of journals in other specialty areas covers epidemiology, cancer, drugs, and analytical chemistry. These journals frequently contain related toxicological material although their scope is broader. The general scientific journals are titles in broad scientific disciplines that often publish articles of toxicologic significance. The newsletters provide currency in select areas of toxicology.

The toxicologist's area of research will dictate what supplemental serials outside those listed here he should become familiar with. Dermatology journals, for instance, are an obviously excellent source of information for skin diseases induced by hazardous substances. Journals in obstetrics and gynecology should be consulted for teratology information. Cancer, epidemiology, and public health are but a few additional specialties to which journals with valuable toxicologic information are devoted. Many of the specialty toxicology journals in the following list began publication in the 1970s. The 1980s is likely to see a continued growth in periodical publication for this subject.

Additional journals may be located in Bowker periodical directories (a,b) and NLM's *SERLINE* file. The Kissman article in the *Information Handling* section of this guide lists journals that are highly cited in the *TOXLINE* file. The Cosmides book in the *Monographs* section provides key journals in areas such as the environment, teratology, mutagenesis, etc. Most of the libraries associated with the institutions in the *Organizations* section have their own lists of periodical holdings and procuring such lists may aid in developing a special collection.

The journal article is probably the form of literature utilized most widely by scientists. This is especially true in toxicology. Research findings may be reported at the earliest stages informally among colleagues and later as meeting papers, but it is via the professional journal that studies are first reported widely.

The newsletters report recent findings and events in a brief journalistic format.

Indexes, abstracts, and bibliographic data bases may need to be accessed before articles can be conveniently located by a wide audience. The followings lists, although focusing on journals that will no doubt be of value to toxicologists, should not become a surrogate for the thousands of other journals that publish potentially relevant articles.

References

(a) *Ulrich's International Periodicals Directory*. New York. RR Bowker. 1932–

(b) *Irregular Serials and Annuals: An International Directory*. New York. RR Bowker. 1967–

Specialty Journals—Toxicology

406. *Acta Pharmacologica et Toxicologica*
Copenhagen. Munksgaard. 1, 1945–

Articles on experimental and clinical toxicology along with experimental pharmacology. Case reports on poisoning are not included.

407. *Advances in Modern Toxicology*
New York. Hemisphere Publication Corporation. 1, 1976–

Monographic series with each volume concentrating on a broad topic and containing review articles. Extensive list of references. Some titles in the series are: *New Concepts in Safety Evaluation* (1, 1976), *Toxicology of Trace Elements* (2, 1977), *Environmental Cancer* (3, 1977), *Dermatotoxicology and Pharmacology* (4, 1977), and *Mutagenesis* (5, 1978).

408. *Advances in the Study of Birth Defects*
Baltimore. University Park Press. 1, 1979–

The first volume in this series discusses teratogenic mechanisms. Volume 2 deals with teratological testing.

409. *American Industrial Hygiene Association Journal*
Akron, Ohio. American Industrial Hygiene Association. 19, 1958–
[Continues *American Industrial Hygiene Association Quarterly*].

Although this journal deals heavily with monitoring and control of exposure and analytical techniques and equipment, and less with health effects per se, there are many articles of relevance expecially in inhalation, heat, noise, and radiation toxicology. Lists meetings, conferences, courses. Book reviews. List of AIHA accredited laboratories appears in each issue. NIOSH Current Intelligence Bulletins are reprinted in this journal. Sections on employment and classified advertising.

410. *Annual Review of Pharmacology and Toxicology*
Palo Alto. Annual Reviews. 16, 1976– [Continues *Annual Review of Pharmacology*]

There is often a prefatory chapter about the life of a distinguished researcher. Each annual has author and subject indexes to the volume along with a cumulative index of contributing authors and list of chapter titles for the 5 most recent volumes. Each volume also contains a Review of Reviews.

411. *Aquatic Toxicology*
Amsterdam. Elsevier/North-Holland. 1, 1981–

Devoted to the mechanisms and assessment of toxicity in aquatic environments, at all levels—from the community to the cellular. Topics such as uptake, metabolism, and excretion are included.

412. *Archives of Environmental Contamination and Toxicology*
New York. Springer Verlag. 1, 1972–

Publishes scientific articles on contaminants in the environment (air, water, soil), the introduction of toxic substances into the environment, and waste.

413. *Archives of Environmental Health*
Washington. Heldref Publications. 1, 1960–

Publishes articles on human health effects of environmental agents. Covers clinical, experimental, and epidemiological studies. Relevant animal studies are also included. Announcements of courses and meetings.

414. *Archives of Toxicology. Archiv für Toxikologie.*
Berlin. Springer Verlag. 32, 1974– [Continues *Archiv für Toxikologie*]

"The 'Archives of Toxicology' accepts Reviews, Original Papers and Short Communications concerned with the observation (case histories), description and experimental investigation of the toxic effects of substances on humans and animals, including methods of treatment or attempted treatment and detection methods in forensic toxicology."

415. *Association of Food and Drug Officials Quarterly*
Littleton, Co. Association of Food and Drug Officials. 41, 1977– [Continues *Quarterly Bulletin—Association of Food and Drug Officials*]

Contains papers presented at various food and drug official meetings.

Emphasis on marketing, management, legislation, regulation, and safety of food and drugs, including potentially toxic ones.

416. *Banbury Report*
Cold Spring Harbor, NY. Cold Spring Harbor Laboratory. 1, 1979–

Consists of an ongoing series of conferences on cancer and biological risk assessment held at the Banbury Center. Each conference results in one bound volume. Some of the titles already published are *Assessing Chemical Mutagens, Mammalian Cell Mutagenesis, A Safe Cigarette, Cancer Incidence in Defined Populations* and *Ethylene Dichloride: A Potential Health Risk.*

417. *Bulletin of Environmental Contamination and Toxicology*
New York. Springer Verlag. 1, 1966–

Rapid communications in the fields of environmental and food contamination and pollution. Ongoing research is presented as brief reports.

418. *Carcinogenesis*
New York. IRL Press. 1, 1980–

Publishes papers and short communications on "carcinogenesis; mutagenesis; factors modifying these processes such as DNA repair, genetics and nutrition; metabolism of carcinogens; the mechanism of action of carcinogens and promoting agents; epidemiological studies; and the formation, detection, identification and quantification of environmental carcinogens."

419. *Carcinogenesis: A Comprehensive Survey*
New York. Raven Press. 1, 1976–

Some of the volumes published include *Polynuclear Aromatic Hydrocarbons, Mechanisms of Tumor Promotion and Carcinogenesis, Nitrofurans,* and *Modifiers of Chemical Carcinogenesis.*

420. *Chemico-Biological Interactions*
Amsterdam. Elsevier. 1, 1969–

Publishes research articles, brief communications, and reviews on effects of chemicals foreign to the organism under consideration. Synthetic and natural exogenous chemicals may include toxins, chemotherapeutic agents, carcinogens, herbicides, pesticides, teratogens, food additives, and pollutants.

421. *Clinical Toxicology*
New York. Marcel Dekker. 1, 1968–

Concentrates on poisoning from a pragmatic viewpoint with many articles on case reports, diagnosis, and treatment. Issues often include editorials, letters to the editor, news items, and announcements.

422. *Clinical Toxicology Consultant*
Memphis. Clinical Toxicology Consultant. 1, 1979–

Provides ''the practicing clinician and other health care providers with up to date information regarding current trends and promising new developments in the prevention, detection, diagnosis, and treatment of acute and chronic toxicities from drugs and environmental chemicals.'' Each issue includes a list of forthcoming articles.

423. *CRC Critical Reviews in Toxicology*
Cleveland. Chemical Rubber Company. 1, 1971–

Lengthy critical evaluations with several hundred references per review not uncommon. The editor of the journal is president of the Chemical Industry Institute of Toxicology (CIIT). In addition to the author and editor, the referee for each article is identified.

424. *CRC Handbook Series in Clinical Laboratory Science. Section B: Toxicology*
West Palm Beach, Florida. Chemical Rubber Company. 1, 1978–

The first volume in this reference handbook series deals with chromatography, immunoassay of drugs, and microcrystal tests. Toxicology is considered from the analytic point of view with detection and identification, qualitative and quantitative, of chemical substances, being of prime concern. There is some text and many tables such as melting points, solubilities of antibiotics, and retention data in chromatographic analyses for assorted classes of data.

425. *Current Intelligence Bulletin—NIOSH*
Cincinnati, Ohio. US Center for Disease Control. 1, 1975–

Each issue is devoted to a given product, chemical, or class of chemicals. A joint effort of NIOSH and OSHA, this bulletin is part of the NIOSH Current Intelligence System, which provides new information on ''occupational hazards that are either unrecognized or are greater than generally known.''

426. *Developments in Toxicology and Environmental Science*
Amsterdam. Elsevier North Holland. 1, 1977–

Some recent titles have been: *Clinical Chemistry and Chemical Toxicology of Metals* (1), *Progress in Genetic Toxicology* (2), *Chemical Toxicology of Food* (3), *Toxicology and Occupational Medicine* (4),

Estrogens in the Environment (5), *The Scientific Basis of Toxicity Assessment* (6), *Progress in Environmental Mutagenesis* (7).

427. *Drug and Chemical Toxicology*
New York. Marcel Dekker. 1, 1977/78–

''... full-length research papers, review articles, and short notes broadly pertaining to animal toxicology, teratology, mutagenesis, and carcinogenesis.''

428. *Drug Metabolism and Disposition: The Biological Fate of Chemicals*
Baltimore. Williams and Wilkins. 1, 1973–

Articles on transformation and fate of chemicals in living systems. A publication of the American Society for Pharmacology and Experimental Therapeutics.

429. *Drug Metabolism Reviews*
New York. Marcel Dekker. 1, 1972–

Publishes critical reviews in areas such as pharmacodynamics, biotransformation, drug metabolites, factors influencing drug metabolism, etc.

430. *Ecotoxicology and Environmental Safety*
New York. Academic Press. 1, June 1977–

Deals with ''studies of the biologic and toxic effects caused by natural or synthetic chemical pollutants to ecosystems, whether animal, plant, or microbial.''

431. *Environmental Health Perspectives*
Research Triangle Park, North Carolina. National Institute of Environmental Health Sciences. 1, 1972–

Concentrates on the effects of the environment on the health of man. Many issues devoted to special topics. These include volumes 1. *PCBs,* 3. *Phthalate Esters,* 5. *Chlorinated dibenzodioxins and dibenzofurans,* 6. *Chemical Mutagenicity Data in Relation to Population Risk,* 7. *Low Level Lead Toxicity,* 8. *Cadmium,* 9. *Asbestos,* 10. *Mobile air emission, Biometerological Hazards,* 11. *Plastics,* 12. *Heavy Metals,* 14. *Insecticides,* 15. *Liver and Kidney,* 16. *Lung,* 17. *Plastics,* 18. *Development,* 19. *Arsenic and Lead,* 21. *Vinyl Chloride,* 22. *Air Pollution, Extrapolation from Animal to Man,* 23. *PCBs,* 24. *Gonads, PCBs,* 25. *Metals,* 26. *Cardiovascular System, Nervous System,* 27. *Plants as Environmental Mutagen Monitors, Hazardous Solid Wastes and their Disposal,* 28. *Cadmium,* 29. *Pollutants and High Risk Groups,* 31.

Aneuploidy, 32. *Statistics and the Environment,* 33. *Intestines, Coal Utilization,* 34. *Aquatic Toxicology, Mineral Fibers and Particulates,* 35. *Pulmonary Research,* 36. *Negative Ionization,* 37. *Pollen Systems.*

432. *Environmental Mutagenesis*
New York. Liss. 1, 1979–

The official journal of the Environmental Mutagen Society. Research papers, book and article reviews, meeting reports, list of papers accepted for publication in future issues. Stresses environmental mutagenesis, genetics, and public health.

433. *Environmental Research*
New York. Academic Press. 1, 1967–

Broadly concerned with environmental biology and medicine. Original research, reviews, and selected book reviews. The editor-in-chief and assistant editors are affiliated with the Environmental Sciences Laboratory of the Mount Sinai School of Medicine. Environmental health is the major thrust of this journal.

434. *Food and Cosmetics Toxicology*
Oxford. Pergamon Press. 1, 1963–

''The Journal is primarily intended for the use of food scientists and technologists, manufacturers, and administrators who neither read nor have access to the medical, pharmacological, or toxicological literature.'' Published for the British Industrial Biological Research Association (BIBRA). The first section of each issue contains research articles with international coverage. Book reviews. General interest articles and abstracts of articles with comments prepared by BIBRA. Announcements of meetings. List of forthcoming papers to appear in next issue. Supplements on special topics published occasionally.

435. *Food, Drug, Cosmetic Law Journal*
Chicago. Commerce Clearing House. 5, 1950– [Continues Food, Drug, Cosmetic Law Quarterly]

Articles on legal concerns relating to food, drugs, and cosmetics and a forum for discussion of general issues in these areas.

436. *Foreign Compound Metabolism in Mammals*
London. The Chemical Society. 1, 1970–

Excellent review articles on xenobiotic metabolism. Drugs, food constituents, agriculturals, and other industrial chemicals are all within the scope of this publication.

437. *Fundamental and Applied Toxicology*
Akron, OH. Society of Toxicology. 1, 1981–

The new official journal of the Society of Toxicology. A professional journal covering the subject broadly and including research in areas such as molecular toxicology, risk assessment, regulatory controls, methods and equipment, aquatic toxicology, environmental toxicology, and safety evaluation.

438. *Hazardous Materials Management Journal*
Germantown, MD. Aspen Systems. 1, 1979–

An outstanding source dealing with regulations, legislation, economics, politics, labor and other societal issues associated with hazardous materials. The articles in the journal often raise important philosophical issues of interest to government, industry, and the public.

439. *Health Physics*
Elmsford, NY. Pergamon Press. 1, 1958–

Scope covers adverse effects of radiation on man and his environment. Original articles, letters, editorials, book reviews, plus international news items in health physics.

440. *International Archives of Occupational and Environmental Health*
Berlin. Springer. 25, 1975– [Continues *Internationales Archiv fur Arbeitsmedizin*]

Publishes reviews, original investigations, short communications, and documents of international meetings. Occupational and ambient problems are the main concerns of this journal. Some foreign language articles.

441. *International Journal of Clinical Pharmacology, Therapy, and Toxicology*
Munich. Dustri-Verlag Feistle. 18, 1980– [Continues *International Journal of Clinical Pharmacology and Biopharmacy*]

Worldwide contributions in areas such as pharmacology, biometrics, metabolism, and clinical toxicology.

442. *International Journal of Radiation Biology and Related Studies in Physics, Chemistry, and Medicine*
London. Taylor and Francis. 1, 1959–

Concentrates on effects of radiation on biological systems.

443. *JOM. Journal of Occupational Medicine*
Chicago. American Occupational Medical Association. 17, 1975–
[Continues *Journal of Occupational Medicine*]

Often publishes epidemiological studies. Carries original articles, letters, reviews.

444. *Journal of Analytical Toxicology*
Niles, Il. Preston Publications. 1, 1977–

Research papers, reviews, short communications, book reviews, on analytical methods relating to toxic substances and their metabolites. Sections on New Products, New Literature Available and a listing of meetings and short courses.

445. *Journal of Applied Toxicology*
Philadelphia, Heyden. 1,1981–

Emphasizes the direct clinical and industrial applications of toxicology. Encompasses such fields as teratology, reproduction, mutagenesis, carcinogenesis, health, the environment, pathology, pharmacokinetics and biological mechanisms. Sections on communications, and letters. Includes a ''toxicology update'' section containing articles which discuss new findings and reviews.

446. *Journal of Environmental Pathology and Toxicology*
Park Forest South, Il. Pathotox Publishers Inc. 1, 1977–

Official organ of the American College of Toxicology. Articles grouped into the following sections (each with its own editors: Environmental Mutagenesis and Genetic Toxicology, Nutritional Toxicology and Pharmacology, Inhalation Toxicology and Pathology, Toxicology and Environmental Health, Dermal Toxicology. Book reviews. Announcements.

447. *Journal of Environmental Science and Health, Part B: Pesticides, Food Contaminants, and Agricultural Wastes.*
New York. Marcel Dekker. 11, 1976– [Continues in part *Environmental Letters*]
Original research reports. Scope includes analytical techniques, metabolism of pesticides, contaminants and wastes, ways of detoxification, and pest control.

448. *Journal of Environmental Science and Health, Part C: Environmental Health Sciences*
New York. Marcel Dekker. 13, 1978– [Continues in part *Environmental Letters*]

Deals with chemicals introduced into the environment. Covered are teratogenesis, mutagenesis, carcinogenesis, and toxicology. ''Emphasis will be placed on biochemical, physiological, behavioral, and pathological alterations.''

449. *Journal of Toxicology and Environmental Health*
Washington. Hemisphere. 1, September 1975–

"Publishes original research papers within the broad fields of toxicology, teratology, environmental toxicology, drug metabolism, carcinogenesis, mutagenesis, and health effects of toxic and environmental factors." Book reviews, announcements. Supplements (a recent one on benzene toxicity).

450. *Modern Pharmacology—Toxicology*
New York. Marcel Dekker. 2, 1975–

A series of monographs and textbooks. Past titles include *Cadmium Toxicity, Body Temperature, Developments in Opiate Research.*

451. *Mutation Research*
Amsterdam. Elsevier. 1, 1964–

Original research, review articles, and short communications "concerning mutagenesis, chromosome breakage and related subjects."

452. *National Clearinghouse for Poison Control Centers Bulletin*
Washington. Public Health Service. 1957–

Contains information on clinical toxicology. Often includes citations from the recent literature.

453. *Neurobehavioral Toxicology*
Fayetville, NY. Ankho International. 1, 1979–

". . . original reports of systematic studies in the areas of neural toxicology and teratology in which the primary emphasis and theoretical context are on the nervous system and behavior."

454. *Neurotoxicology*
Park Forest, IL. Pathotox. 1, 1979–

Papers deal with the effects of poisonous substances on the nervous system of man or animal. Environmental chemicals are emphasized but drugs and other natural compounds are also in scope. Announcements, Book Reviews, and Abstracts of Meetings are periodically published.

455. *Neurotoxicology*
New York. Raven Press. 1, 1977–

Volume 1 of this title is divided into the following chapters: tranquilizers, narcotics and anesthetics, stimulants, antidepressants, and hallucinogens, heavy and trace metals; antimicrobials; industrial chemicals; pesticides; anorexic agents; and pathogenic considerations in neurotoxicology. A subject index is included.

456. *Pesticide Biochemistry and Physiology*
New York. Academic Press. 1, 1971–

Original research published in insecticides, fungicides, rodenticides, herbicides, acaricides, nematocides, and related compounds. Biochemical and physiological effects of these substances in target and nontarget organisms, as well as metabolism of the agents themselves are topics considered.

457. *Pesticides Monitoring Journal*
Chamblee, GA. Environmental Protection Agency. 1, 1967–

Provides information on levels of pesticides relative to humans and their environment.

458. *Progress in Chemical Toxicology*
New York. Academic Press. 1, 1963–

Series of review articles in chemical toxicology.

459. *Radiation Research*
New York. Academic Press. 1, 1954–

The official organ of the Radiation Research Society. Publishes "original articles dealing with radiation effects and related subjects in areas of physics, chemistry, biology, and medicine. The term 'radiation' is used in its broadest sense and includes specifically ionizing radiation, ultraviolet, visible, and infrared light as well as microwaves, ultrasound and heat."

460. *Registry of Toxic Effects of Chemical Substances (RTECS)*
Rockville, MD. NIOSH. 1975– [Continues *Toxic Substances List*]

The publication of known toxic substances is a NIOSH mandate. Presents basic toxicity information and other data for chemicals. 5 Indexes—Complete File Index, Carcinogenic and Neoplastigenic Citations Index, Teratogenic Citations Index, Mutagenic Citations Index, and Human Effects Citation Index. Trade names and mixtures are excluded. Data appearing includes prime name, CAS Registry Number, molecular weight, molecular formula, synonyms, toxic dose date, cited references, and reviews, standards and regulations, NIOSH Criteria Documents and NCI status. Available in hard copy, fiche, and on-line from NLM.

461. *Residue Reviews*
New York. Springer Verlag. 1, 1962–

Critical reviews on the introduction of foreign chemicals into the environment. Pesticides, food additives and other contaminant chemicals are within the scope of this journal. Subject index in each volume.

462. *Reviews in Biochemical Toxicology*
New York. Elsevier North Holland. 1, 1979–

The editors of this review series are from North Carolina State University and NIEHS. Broad topics covered in the first volume include xenobiotic-metabolizing enzymes, biochemical toxicology of organs and organ-systems, toxic compounds, modes of toxic action, and methodology of biochemical toxicology.

463. *Rochester International Conference on Environmental Toxicity*
NY. Raven Press. 3, 1970– [Continues *Rochester Conference on Environmental Toxicity*]

Papers and discussion from one of the world's major conferences in environmental toxicology.

464. *Scandinavian Journal of Work, Environment, and Health*
Helsinki. Occupational Health Foundation, Finland. 1, 1975–

Articles on environmental and work-related exposures. Letters to the editor, announcements, book reviews. Published jointly by the National Board of Occupational Safety and Health, Sweden; the Institute of Occupational Health, Finland; the Swedish Medical Society, Section for Environmental Health, Sweden; the Work Research Institutes, Norway; the Working Environment Fund, Denmark.

465. *Side Effects of Drugs Annual*
Amsterdam. Excerpta Medica. 1, 1977–

Provides "a critical and up-to-date account of new information relating to adverse drug reactions and interactions from the clinician's point of view." The indexes to these annuals are cumulated over limited time periods.

466. *Teratogenesis, Carcinogenesis and Mutagenesis*
New York. Alan R. Liss. 1, 1980–

From the editorial of the inaugural issue: ". . . one would anticipate considerable overlap between agents that are teratogenic, mutagenic, or carcinogenic . . . the major purpose of the journal is to foster interactions among investigators in the fields of teratogenesis, carcinogenesis, and mutagenesis. We especially welcome papers that will deepen our understanding of the similarities and dissimilarities of these fields; manuscripts that describe methods for characterizing agents that induce adverse effects; and reports of basic research."

467. *Teratology*
Philadelphia. Wistar Institute of Anatomy and Biology. 1, 1968–

Deals with all aspects of abnormal development. Publishes original reports, letters, "Teratogen Update" (a feature on current information on identified human teratogens). Sections of journal are Clinical Teratology, Experimental Teratology, Genetics and Cytogenetics, Epidemiology, Fetal Pharmacology, and Behavioral Teratology.

468. *Topics in Environmental Health*
Amsterdam. Elsevier/North-Holland. 1,1978–

Recent volumes include *The Biogeochemistry of lead in the environment* and *The chemistry, biochemistry and biology of cadmium.*

469. *Toxicologic Pathology*
Newark, Delaware. Society of Toxicologic Pathologists. 1978–
[Continues *Bulletin of the Society of Pharmacological and Environmental Pathologists*]

The official journal of the Society of Toxicologic Pathologists. Publishes articles on pathology as it relates to pharmacological, chemical, and environmental agents.

470. *Toxicological and Environmental Chemistry Reviews*
New York. Gordon and Breach. 1, 1972–

"International journal devoted to fundamental aspects of analysis, environmental fate, metabolism, and effects of chemicals both of synthetic and natural origin as related to environment and human health."

471. *Toxicological European Research. Recherche Europeene en Toxicologie*
Puteaux. Editions Ouranos. 1, 1978– [Supersedes *European Journal of Toxicology and Environmental Hygiene. Journal Europeen de Toxicologie*]

Articles in English, French, and German on toxicology, the environment and legal matters.

472. *Toxicology*
Amsterdam. Elsevier. 1, 1973–

The broad scope of the journal is evident in its subtitle, "An international journal concerned with the effects of chemicals on living systems."

473. *Toxicology Annual*
New York. Marcel Dekker. 1, 1974–

Review articles covering toxicology broadly. Topics include veterinary, preventive, forensic, analytical, and clinical toxicology. Section of free communications.

474. *Toxicology and Applied Pharmacology*
New York. Academic Press. 1, 1959–

Primarily original scientific research. Also short reviews, communications, announcements and letters. In addition to subject and author indexes, each volume has a chemical index. Articles "pertaining to alterations in tissue structure or function resulting from the administration of chemicals, drugs, or natural products to animal or man." Supplements are published.

475. *Toxicology Letters*
Amsterdam. Elsevier. 1 July 1977–

Provides for rapid publication of short papers on all areas of toxicological research. International in scope.

476. *Toxicon*
Oxford. Pergamon Press. 1, 1962–

The official journal of the International Society on Toxinology. Subtitle is "An international journal devoted to the exchange of knowledge on the poisons derived from animals, plants and microorganisms." Publishes supplements, the first being an 1100 page volume consisting of the proceedings of a symposium on animal, plant and microbial toxins.

477. *Toxics Control Series*
Washington. Government Institutes. 1977–

Consists of the proceedings of the annual Toxic Control Conferences sponsored by Government Institutes. Recent themes have been "Implementing the Regulatory Program" and "Toxic Control in the 80's."

478. *Trace Substances in Environmental Health*
Columbia, MO. University of Missouri. 1, 1967–

Consists of proceedings of the University of Missouri's Annual Conferences on Trace Substances in Environmental Health, the purposes being "to explore the biological, economical and health significances of the numerous inorganic and organic substances which are present, normally, in trace amounts in our environment, particularly in our air, food, and water."

479. *Veterinary and Human Toxicology*
Kansas. American College of Veterinary Toxicologists. 19, 1977–
[Continues *Veterinary Toxicology*].

Covers the "broad field of toxicology, including news items and announcements, manuscripts of original research, scientific reviews, and field observations in domestic and wild animals or man." Book reviews, meeting abstracts, job opportunities, and forthcoming meetings.

Specialty Journals—Related Areas

480. *Advances in Pharmacology and Chemotherapy*
New York. Academic Press. 7, 1969–
[Union of *Advances in Pharmacology* and *Advances in Chemotherapy*]

481. *American Journal of Epidemiology*
Baltimore. School of Hygiene and Public Health of Johns Hopkins University. 81, 1965– [Continues *American Journal of Hygiene*]

482. *British Journal of Cancer*
London. HK Lewis. 1, 1947–

483. *Cancer Research*
Baltimore. Waverly Press. 1, 1941–

484. *Clinical Pharmacology and Drug Epidemiology*
New York. ADIS Press. 1, 1976–

485. *Clinical Pharmacology and Therapeutics*
St. Louis. Mosby. 1, 1960–

486. *Clinical Pharmacokinetics*
New York. ADIS Press. 1, 1976–

487. *Epidemiologic Reviews*
Baltimore. Johns Hopkins University Press. 1, 1979–

488. *Fate of Drugs in the Organism*
New York. Marcel Dekker. 1, 1974–

489. *International Journal of Environmental Analytical Chemistry*
London. Gordon and Breach. 1, 1971–

490. *International Journal of Epidemiology*
London. Oxford University Press. 1, 1972–

491. *JNCI. Journal of the National Cancer Institute*
Bethesda, MD. National Cancer Institute. 1, 1940–

492. *Journal of Pharmacokinetics and Biopharmaceutics*
New York. Plenum. 1, 1973–

493. *Journal of Pharmacology and Experimental Therapeutics*
Baltimore. Williams and Wilkins. 1, 1909–

494. *Molecular Pharmacology*
New York, Academic Press. 1, 1965–

495. *Pharmacological Reviews*
Baltimore. Williams and Wilkins. 1, 1949–

General Scientific Journals

496. *Annals of the New York Academy of Sciences*
New York. New York Academy of Sciences. 1, 1877–

497. *British Medical Journal*
London. British Medical Association. 1857–

498. *JAMA. Journal of the American Medical Association*
Chicago. American Medical Association. 173, 1960– [Continues *Journal of the American Medical Association*]

499. *Lancet*
London. Lancet. 1823–

500. *Nature*
London. Macmillan Journals. 1, 1869–

501. *Proceedings of the National Academy of Sciences of the United States of America*
Washington. National Academy of Sciences. 1, 1915–

502. *Science*
Washington. American Association for the Advancement of Science. 1, 1883–

503. *World Health Organization (WHO) Technical Report Series*
Geneva. World Health Organization. 1, 1950–

Newsletters

504. *BIBRA Bulletin*
Carshalton, England. British Industrial Research Association.

News, review articles, abstracts, book reviews. Keeps current on international legislation and world news.

505. *Chemical Regulation Reporter*
Washington, DC. Bureau of National Affairs

Very current information on news about and regulation of chemicals.

506. *Environmental Health Letter*
Washington. Gershon W. Fishbein

A newsletter concentrating on government, industry, legislation, regulations. Keeps you up-to-date on EPA's activities.

507. *Environment Report*
Washington. Trends Publishing. 1, 1970–

Reports news and trends in environmental matters.

508. *Food Chemical News*
Washington. Food Chemical News. 1, 1959–

"Regulation of food additives, colors, pesticides, and allied products."

509. *Food and Drug Letter*
Washington. Washington Business Information. 1, 1976–

Regulations, marketing, legislation.

510. *Industrial Hygiene News Report*
Chicago. Flournoy and Associates. 1, 1958–

"Reporting on new methodology and research in the recognition, evaluation, and control of workplace hazards."

511. *IRPTC Bulletin*
Geneva. International Register of Potentially Toxic Chemicals. 1, 1977–

The one essential periodical for keeping current with toxicology activities internationally. Provides valuable information on foreign organizations, legislation, and information gathering.

512. *Newsletter. Forum for the Advancement of Toxicology*
Memphis, TN. Forum for the Advancement of Toxicology.

The Forum is an informal group of professionals interested in advancing the field of toxicology.

513. *Occupational Health and Safety Letter*
Washington. Gershon W. Fishbein.

Legislation and regulations. Keeps the reader informed on activities of NIOSH and OSHA.

514. *Toxic Materials News*
Silver Spring, MD. Business Publishers.

News primarily about government regulatory agencies and legislation involving toxic substances.

Chapter 8

Audiovisuals

There are, as yet, only a limited number of audiovisuals in toxicology. Audiovisuals are especially useful as instructional tools and in demonstrating methods and procedures. I have not viewed the audiovisuals and they are, therefore, not annotated. Additional sources to consult for audiovisuals are NLM's *Audiovisuals Catalog* (a), *National Medical Audiovisual Center Catalog* (b), and other health sciences audiovisuals catalogs (c,d,e,f). The library or public information office of most of the agencies involved in toxicology may also have available lists of organizationally produced audiovisuals.

References

(a) *National Library of Medicine Audiovisuals Catalog*. Bethesda, MD. United States Department of Health, Education, and Welfare, National Library of Medicine. 1977–

(b) *National Medical Audiovisual Center Catalog*. Atlanta. National Medical Audiovisual Center. 1968–

(c) National Information Center for Educational Media. *Index to health and safety education,* 3rd ed. Los Angeles. University of Southern California. 1977.

(d) *The Videolog: Programs for the Health Sciences*. New York. Esselte Video. 1979–

(e) *Medical Catalog of Selected Audiovisual Materials Produced by the United States Government*. Washington, DC. National Audiovisual Center, National Archives and Records Service. 1980.

(f) *Index to Audiovisual Serials in the Health Sciences*. Chicago. Medical Library Association. 1, 1977–

515. *Accidental poisoning in children*
 [Videorecording]
 Tubergen DG
 Ann Arbor. University of Michigan Medical Center. 1973

516. *Additives and hyperactivity*
 [Sound recording]
 Feingold BF
 New York. Huxley Institute for Biosocial Research. 1978.

517. *Biological effects of ionizing radiation*
 [Videorecording]
 Barnett MH
 Rockville, MD. Training Productions Center, Bureau of Radiological
 Health. 1977.

518. *Carcinogenesis: A perspective*
 [Videorecording]
 Rawson RW
 Houston. University of Texas System Cancer Center, M.D. Anderson
 Hospital and Tumor Institute. 1976.

519. *Carcinogenic anesthetics: A key to cancer prevention*
 [Videorecording]
 Poel WE
 Houston. University of Texas System Cancer Center, M.D. Anderson
 Hospital and Tumor Institute. 1977.

520. *Chemical carcinogenesis: The staging theory*
 [Videorecording]
 Pedersen ML
 Berkeley, CA. Regents of the University of California. 1979.

521. *Clastogenic effects of carcinogens*
 [Videorecording]
 Altenburg LC
 Houston. University of Texas System Cancer Center, M.D. Anderson
 Hospital and Tumor Institute. 1976.

522. *Coal workers' pneumoconiosis*
 [Slides and audiocassette]
 Wismar BL
 New York. American Lung Association for the American Thoracic So-
 ciety. 1976.

523. *Considerations of benzo(a)pyrene metabolism and carcinogenicity*

[Videorecording]
Thomas B
Houston. University of Texas System Cancer Center, M.D. Anderson
Hospital and Tumor Institute. 1976.

524. *Drug metabolism*
[Videorecording]
Ayerst Medical Information Service
New York. Ayerst Laboratories. 1978.

525. *Drugs: action and interaction*
[Filmstrip]
Concept Media
Costa Mesa, CA. Concept Media. 1976.

526. *Effects of ionizing radiation on mammalian DNA*
[Videorecording]
Shanka F
Houston. University of Texas System Cancer Center, M.D. Anderson
Hospital and Tumor Institute. 1975.

527. *Gastric lavage*
[Videorecording]
American College of Physicians
Philadelphia. American College of Physicians. 1976.

528. *Hepatocarcinogens: The relation of structure to carcinogenic activity*
[Videorecording]
Kadlubar F
Houston. University of Texas System Cancer Center, M.D. Anderson
Hospital and Tumor Institute. 1976.

529. *How to manage acute poisoning and overdose*
[Sound recording]
Rumack BH
Chicago. Teach'em, Inc. 1977.

530. *Lead poisoning*
[Slides and audiocassette]
Gerrick DJ
Lorain, OH. Dayton Lab. 1979.

531. *Lead poisoning*
[Videorecording]
Balcerzak SP

Columbus, OH. Ohio State University, Medical Audiovisual and Television Center. 1971.

532. *Long term effects of ionizing radiation exposure*
[Videorecording]
Barnett MH
Rockville, MD. Training Productions Center, Bureau of Radiological Health. 1977.

533. *Lung vs. the environment, The*
[Slides and audiocassette]
Sanchis JV, Newhouse MT
Hamilton, Ontario. Mcmaster University, Health Sciences. 1976.

534. *Management of acute poisoning*
[Sound recording]
Rumack BH
Chicago. Teach'em, Inc. 1977.

535. *Medical effects of the atomic bomb*
[Motion picture]
U.S. Department of the Army
Washington. U.S. Department of the Army. 1950.

536. *Membrane involvement in chemical carcinogenesis*
[Videorecording]
Walborg E
Houston. University of Texas System Cancer Center, M.D. Anderson Hospital and Tumor Institute. 1976.

537. *Metabolism of carcinogens*
[Videorecording]
Strobel HW
Houston. University of Texas System Cancer Center, M.D. Anderson Hospital and Tumor Institute. 1976.

538. *Mercury poisoning in man*
[Slides and audiocassette]
Gerrick DJ
Lorain, OH. Dayton Lab. 1979.

539. *Mislabeled and unlabeled deaths*
[Videorecording]
Helpern M
New York. New York University Medical Center. 1978.

540. *Mutagenic activity of carcinogens*
[Videorecording]
Matney TS
Houston. University of Texas System Cancer Center, M.D. Anderson
Hospital and Tumor Institute. 1976.

541. *Mutagenicity of vinyl chloride metabolites and related compounds*
[Videorecording]
Laumbach A
Houston. University of Texas System Cancer Center, M.D. Anderson
Hospital and Tumor Institute. 1976.

542. *Mutagen testing*
[Videorecording]
Legator MS
Houston. University of Texas System Cancer Center, M.D. Anderson
Hospital and Tumor Institute. 1976.

543. *Mutational model for carcinogenesis, A*
[Videorecording]
Knudson AG
Houston. University of Texas System Cancer Center, M.D. Anderson
Hospital and Tumor Institute. 1976.

544. *Noise and hearing loss*
[Videorecording]
Henderson D, Alberti PW
Rochester, Minn. American Academy of Ophthalmology and Otolaryn-
gology. 1976.

545. *Occupational and ocular effects of microwaves*
[Videorecording]
Hirsch S
Rockville, MD. Bureau of Radiological Health. 1977.

546. *Occupational dermatoses*
[Videorecording]
Birmingham DJ
Rockville, MD. National Institute for Occupational Safety and Health,
U.S. Department of Health, Education, and Welfare. 1973.

547. *Organophosphate pesticide poisonings*
[Motion picture]
U.S. Environmental Protection Agency
Washington. U.S. Environmental Protection Agency, Office of Pes-
ticide Programs. 1969.

548. *Pesticide poisonings and injuries*
[Slides and audiocassette]
Morgan DP
Oakdale, Iowa. Institute of Agricultural Medicine and Environmental health, Department of Preventive Medicine and Environmental Health, College of Medicine, University of Iowa, 1978.

549. *Poison hazards in the home*
[Videorecording]
Rauber AP
Atlanta. Georgia Regional Medical Television Network. 1977.

550. *Poison plants: Dangerous plants around us*
[Videorecording]
Rauber AP
Atlanta. Georgia Regional Medical Television Network. 1976.

551. *Population dose and health impact of the Three Mile Island accident*
[Videorecording]
Christopher N
Rockville, MD. Bureau of Radiological Health. 1979.

552. *Principles of pharmacokinetics*
[Videorecording]
Lipicky RJ
Bethesda, MD. U.S. Department of Health, Education, and Welfare, Public Health Service, National Institutes of Health. 1978.

553. *Salmonella-microsome mutagenicity test*
[Videorecording]
Ames BN
Berkeley. University of California. 1976.

554. *Survey of environmental carcinogens*
[Videorecording]
Griffin AC
Houston. University of Texas System Cancer Center, M.D. Anderson Hospital and Tumor Institute. 1976.

555. *Toxicity of local anesthetic agents*
[Videorecording]
Mendenhall MK
Fort Sam Houston, TX. Academy of Health Sciences. 1974.

556. *Toxicology*
[Videorecording]

Slovis TL, Comerci GD
Tucson. Medical Audiovisual Center, Arizona Medical Center. 1974.

557. *Toxicology of cholinesterase-inhibiting insecticides*
[Slides and audiocassette]
Morgan DP
Oakdale, Iowa. Institute of Agricultural Medicine and Environmental
Health, Department of Preventive Medicine and Environmental Health,
College of Medicine, University of Iowa. 1978.

558. *Toxicology of commonly used herbicides*
[Slides and audiocassette]
Morgan DP
Oakdale, Iowa. Institute of Agricultural Medicine and Environmental
Health, Department of Preventive Medicine and Environmental Health,
College of Medicine, University of Iowa. 1978.

559. *Toxicology of fungicides, rodenticides, and fumigants*
[Slides and audiocassette]
Morgan DP
Oakdale, Iowa. Institute of Agricultural Medicine and Environmental
Health, Department of Preventive Medicine and Environmental Health,
College of Medicine, University of Iowa. 1978.

560. *Ultraviolet light induced carcinogenesis*
[Videorecording]
Black H
Houston. University of Texas System Cancer Center, M.D. Anderson
Hospital and Tumor Institute. 1976.

561. *Vinyl chloride carcinogenesis*
[Videorecording]
Tamburro C
Houston. University of Texas System Cancer Center, M.D. Anderson
Hospital and Tumor Institute. 1976.

562. *What emergency and poison control staff should know about insect stings*
[Sound recording]
Frazier CA
Chicago. Teach'em Inc. 1977.

563. *X-Rays and other modern hazards: diet soda, flame retardant pajamas and
X-Rays: How do risks compare?*
[Videorecording]
Barnett MH
Rockville, MD. Bureau of Radiological Health. 1977.

Chapter 9

Microforms and Card Files

The following services contain primarily product information. They are useful for poison ingredient and treatment data. Physicians treating acute poisoning victims, as well as drug information and poison control centers should derive the most benefit from these tools.

564. *National Clearinghouse for Poison Control Center Cards*
FDA Burea of Drugs, Division of Poison Control HFD-240 5401 Westbard Avenue, Bethesda, MD 20016

Provided to poison control centers, these cards describe products giving ingredient information, toxicity, symptoms and findings, and treatment.

565. *Poisindex*
Micromedex, Inc., Englewood, Colorado 80110

Computer generated microfiche system consisting of product formulation information and poison management treatment information. Micromedex also publishes "Drugdex" and the DeHaen products on drugs.

566. *Toxifile*
Chicago Micro Corporation, Chicago, Illinois 60625

Product ingredient and treatment information. The entire FDA National Clearinghouse for Poison Control Centers computer data base is part of Toxifile.

Chapter 10

Abstracts, Indexes, and Current Awareness

These publications provide access to the literature and, sometimes, summaries of it. The literature cited is usually journal articles although increasingly these tools are devoting space to indexing monographs, technical reports, and other forms of literature. Access is usually by author and subject, as a minimum. Author indexes allow precise verification of a citation if the author and date of an article are known. Subject indexes may be used for the compilation of bibliographies, as well as to scan a subject area for articles of interest.

Major abstracts and indexes are now being published in paper simultaneously with the production of computer tapes and microforms. A separate section of this book is devoted to computer data bases.

Hard copy indexes and/or data bases are the sources used by the toxicology researcher in performing a literature search. They are the most efficient means of tracking down primary literature. Because of the time required to prepare an abstracting or indexing tool (both the intellectual effort of indexing and the effort involved in publication) there is usually an unavoidable and unfortunate lag between the time journal articles appear and the time they are indexed. Current awareness tools published much more rapidly and frequently overcome this to a certain extent as do certain data bases. If on-line journals ever become a reality on a large scale, this problem will be overcome.

Core

567. *Abstracts on Health Effects of Environmental Pollutants*
Philadelphia. Biosciences Information Service of Biological Abstracts. 1, 1972–

Abstracts are drawn from *Biological Abstracts* and citations from *Bioresearch Index*. Subtitle is ''In air, soil and water caused by noise, vibration, radiation, thermal effects, toxic substances for agriculture, industry, research."

568. *CA Selects*
Columbus, Ohio. Chemical Abstracts Service.

A current-awareness publication, this is a series of 76 titles each on a special topic in chemistry. Frequency is once every two weeks and issues consist of abstracts drawn from a search of Chemical Abstracts. Some of the titles more relevant to toxicology are "Chemical Hazards," "Drug and Cosmetic Toxicity," "Food Toxicity," "Carcinogens, Mutagens, and Teratogens," "Environmental Pollution."

569. *Chemical Mutagenesis*
Oak Ridge, Tenn. Oak Ridge National Laboratory. 1971–

Collections of chemical mutagenesis citations for specific years. Indexed by test organism, chemical synonyms, CAS registry number, and cell cultures when applicable. Author index.

570. *Clin-Alert*
Louisville, Kentucky. Science Editors, Inc. 1962–

A biweekly of abstracts on iatrogenic reactions.

571. *Environment Abstracts*
New York. Environment Information Center. 4, 1974– [Continues *Environment Information Access*]

Articles are classified by 21 review categories such as "chemical and biological contamination," "energy," "food and drugs," "noise," "radiological contamination," and "solid waste." Abstracts include information on graphs, drawings, photos, tables, and references. Indexes by subject, industry (e.g., pesticides, organic chemicals), source (i.e., journal title) and author. The Environment Information Center's "Documents on Demand" system allows for dispatch of fiche or hard copy of full articles.

572. *Environment Index, The*
New York. Environment Information Center. 1971–

A major subject index to the environment with geographic and author indexes included. Special features include reviews of environmental issues, legislation, and Environmental Impact Statements for the preceding year. Selections of books, films, periodicals, and major conferences on environmental topics.

573. *Excerpta Medica*
Amsterdam. Excerpta Medica.

This series of international abstracts is arranged by a fairly detailed classification scheme with an augmented subject index. The following titles may be particularly useful in toxicology: "Cancer," "Developmental Biology and Teratology," "Environmental Health and Pollution Control," "Occupational Health and Industrial Medicine," "Pharmacology and Toxicology." Also "Adverse Reactions Titles," an index.

574. *FDA Clinical Experience Abstracts*
Washington. Food and Drug Administration. 15, 1966– [Continues *MLB Journal of Literature Abstracts*].

Covers 180 international biomedical periodicals, primarily in clinical medicine. Treats adverse effects of drugs, cosmetics, household chemicals, pesticides, and food additives. Arranged on index cards which can be separated and filed.

575. *ICRDB Cancergram*
Bethesda, MD. National Cancer Institute.

About 20 titles dealing with chemical, environmental, and radiation carcinogenesis. representative titles are "Radiation Carcinogenesis," "Organ Site Carcinogenesis—Respiratory Tract," "Hormonal Carcinogenesis." This abstracting tool is updated every few weeks and available from NTIS. ICRDB (International Cancer Research Data Bank) is a program of the National Cancer Institute.

576. *Industrial Hygiene Digest*
Pittsburgh. Industrial Health Foundation, Inc. 1, 1937–

Abstracts on all aspects of industrial hygiene.

577. *Pesticides Abstracts*
Washington. Technical Services Division of the Office of Pesticide Programs, Environmental Protection Agency. 7, 1974– [Continues *Health Aspects of Pesticides, Abstract Bulletin*]

Effects of pesticides with regard to monitoring and residues, epidemiology, prevention and treatment, toxicology and pharmacology, and analysis.

578. *Pollution Abstracts*
Louisville, KY. Data Courier. 1, 1970–
Abstracts on "air pollution, marine and freshwater pollution, sewage and wastewater treatment, solid wastes, pesticides and chemical contaminants, noise pollution, radiation, land pollution, and environmental policies, programs, legislation, and education." Subject and author indexes.

579. *Teratology Lookout*
Stockholm. Karolinska Institutet.

References to articles from MEDLARS, Chemical Abstracts and BIOSIS. References show source from which citation was taken. Arranged by broad subject categories.

580. *Toxicology Abstracts*
London. Information Retrieval Ltd. 1, 1978–

Abstracts are grouped into broad classes of substances (e.g., pharmaceuticals, food additives, agrochemicals, industrial chemicals, etc.) Also included is radiation, methodology, legislation, abstracts of reviews and books plus notification of proceedings.

581. *Toxicology Research Projects Directory*
Bethesda, MD. Toxicology Information Subcommittee of the DHEW Committee to Coordinate Toxicology and Related Programs. 1, 1976– (Available from National Technical Information Service, Springfield, VA)

Abstracts of research activities in toxicology and related fields taken from files of the Smithsonian Science Information Exchange. Researchers' names and addresses are provided as is the supporting agency. Bibliographic references may be included. Amount of funds is provided when available. The following indexes are available: subject, investigator, performing organization, supporting agency, master grant number.

582. *TOX/TIPS*
Bethesda, MD. US Toxicology Information Program, National Library of Medicine. June 1976–

Abstracts of research projects on "all areas of long-term testing, as well as epidemiology to determine toxicity." Funding and administrative details are included when available. There are indexes to institutions, investigators and compounds tested. Selective references related to each project have been retrieved from searches of NLM's on-line files.

Supplementary/General

583. *Bibliography of Agriculture*
Phoenix. Oryx Press. 1, 1942–

Created with data provided by the National Agricultural Library of the USDA. Geographic, corporate author, personal author, and subject indexes. Journal articles, government documents, pamphlets, proceedings, etc., are included. Excellent source for toxicology related to food, biotoxins, pesticides, and general environmental pollution.

584. *Biological Abstracts*
Philadelphia. Biosciences Information Service of Biological Abstracts. 1, 1926–

Covers the biological literature. Sections of interest to the toxicologist include Pesticides, Pharmacology, Public Health, Radiation Biology, and Toxicology. Toxicology information is also spread throughout other sections. Excellent access is provided by an author index, a biosystematic index (arranged by taxonomic groups), a generic index (arranged by genus-species names), a concept index (arranged by broad subject concepts) and a subject index (organized by specific keywords). The concept index provides the following breakdowns for toxicology— antidotes and prevention, environmental and industrial, foods, food residues, additives, preservative, general, methods, experimental, pharmacological, veterinary.

585. *Biological Abstracts/RRM*
Philadelphia. Biosciences Information Service. 18, 1980– [Continues *Bioresearch Index*]

Indexes nonjournal literature such as reports, reviews, meetings. Includes synopses of recent life sciences books. Same indexes as in *Biological Abstracts*.

586. *Biological and Agricultural Index*
Bronx, NY. HW Wilson. 19, 1965– [Continues *Agriculture Index*]

"A cumulative subject index to periodicals in the fields of biology, agriculture and related sciences."

587. *Chemical Abstracts*
Columbus, OH. Chemical Abstracts Service. 1907–

Provides broad coverage of chemistry and other sciences. Abstract sections of special interest to toxicology are 1 Pharmacodynamics, 3 Biochemical Interactions, 4 Toxicology, 5 Agrochemicals, and 6 Radiation Biochemistry. Keywork, numerical patent, and author indexes, plus patent concordance.

588. *Current Contents*
Philadelphia. Institute for Scientific Information.

Series of current awareness tools published weekly which reproduce, in a timely fashion, the tables of contents of journals in specialty areas. Among the Current Contents series published are 1 Agriculture, biology, and environmental sciences; 2 Clinical practice; 3 Engineering, technology, and applied sciences; 4 Life sciences; 5 Physical, chemical, and earth sciences; 6 Social and behavioral sciences.

589. *Government Reports Announcements*
Springfield, VA. National Technical Information Service. 75, 1975– [formed by the union of *Government Reports Announcements* and *Government Reports Index*]

Indexes and abstracts technical reports. Indexes by subject, personal author, corporate author, contract number, and accession number. Arranged by 22 NTIS COSATI subject fields. Ones of particular relevance to toxicology are agriculture, bilogical and medical sciences, chemistry, earth sciences and oceanography, energy conversion, and nuclear science and technology.

590. *Index Medicus*
Bethesda, MD. National Library of Medicine. 1, 1960–

One of the major biomedical indexes. Contains citations from nearly 3000 indexed journals and selected monographs. Subject and author indexes. Subject indexes are categorized by NLM's MESH (Medical Subject Headings) classification. 3 useful subheadings which may be applied to certain of the main subject headings and which facilitate toxicological type searching are "adverse effects," "poisoning," and "toxicity."

591. *Monthly Catalogue of United States Government Publications*
Washington. Government Printing Office.

Arranged by agency, this is a good source for locating publications by the Agriculture Department, EPA, OSHA, etc. Most materials listed may be ordered via GPO (Government Printing Office). Author, titles, subject, series, stock number, and keyword indexes. There is also a serials supplement to the monthly catalog which compiles publications issued 3 or more times a year and a select group of annuals and monographic series. This supplement is issued annually.

592. *Science Citation Index*
Philadelphia. Institute for Scientific Information. 1961–

Multidisciplinary index to scientific literature. Includes medicine, agriculture, technology and the behavioral sciences. Journal articles, proceedings, symposia, monographic series and multiauthored books are indexed. Author ("Source") and Subject ("Permuterm Subject") indexes. Unique feature is the Citation Index, which allows for retrieval of literature within a given year, which cites a known item. Premise behind this approach is that an article which has been cited in other articles is somehow related to them in terms of subject matter.

See also:

Ross S, ed. *Toxic Substances Sourcebook* [under *Legislative, Regulatory, and Societal Issues*]

Toxic Substances Sourcebook 2. [under *Legislative, Regulatory, and Societal Issues*]

Chapter 11

Data Bases

One of the most dramatic recent changes in the means of accessing information has been the development of on-line interactive computer data base systems. The computer, through a trained intermediary, is able to coordinate a large number of concepts, manipulate the data, and generate output in a variety of formats.

A distinction is usually made between bibliographic and nonbibliographic data bases (occasionally referred to as data banks, factual data bases, or knowledge banks). Bibliographic data bases, such as MEDLINE and TOXLINE, consist of references to literature. The type of literature varies with the particular data base. Some possible formats of literature cited are journal articles, monographs, technical reports, audiovisuals, research projects, and meeting abstracts. For a journal article, for instance, a data base record will typically contain information such as the author(s) of the article, the title of the article, the title of the journal in which it appears, the volume, number, pages, and date of the issue of the journal in which the article appears. Some data bases offer the convenience of abstracts online and there has even been experimentation with the complete texts of journal articles on-line. Data bases may be used to verify citations, retrieve literature by authors and perhaps most often to retrieve citations on a particular subject. Nonbibliographic data bases contain more of what the scientist would consider true "data" (numeric values) and factual information, often culled from journal articles and handbooks. Examples of information that may be found in nonbibliographic data bases are chemical names and synonyms, LD50s, aquatic toxicity values, threshold limit values, etc. The ease and efficiency of preparing custom-made bibliographies in a variety of complex subjects is possible only because of the speed and processing abilities of modern computers.

Toxicology is fortunate in being a discipline for which a number of specialized data bases exist. In addition, toxicology information is distributed among more general scientific data bases. This spread of information, however, can be perplexing in choosing the right combination of data bases to search. A complete literature search should always be undertaken prior to the initiation of any toxicology search.

Various organizations are responsible for the functioning of data bases. "Producers" create the data bases. "Suppliers" make the data base available to users. "Producers" and "suppliers" may or may not be the same organization. Many producers make the computer tapes themselves available to organizations which then mount them on their own computers. The data bases listed include information on "suppliers," "producers," or other contact.

The data bases listed is a very small sampling of those believed to be most relevant to toxicology. Specialized data bases on food, water, engineering, management, technical reports, newspapers, etc. may also be worth accessing. Some excellent sources for additional detailed information about the data bases listed and the many more specialized ones not included here are Williams' *Computer-Readable Data Bases* (a) and other reference tools (b,c). Various training aids and manuals are also available from data base suppliers. Some of the major suppliers of data bases related to toxicology are as follows:

   I. Bibliographic Retrieval Services, Inc. (BRS)
      Corporation Park
      Building 702
      Scotia, NY 12302

  II. Interactive Sciences Corporation
      918 16th Street NW, Suite 500
      Washington, DC 20006

 III. Lockheed Information Systems
      Dept. 52-08, Bldg. 21
      3251 Hanover Street
      Palo Alto, CA 94304

  IV. National Library of Medicine (NLM)
      8600 Rockville Pike
      Bethesda, MD 20209

   V. Sigma Data Computing Corporation
      2021 K Street, Suite 207
      Washington, DC 20006

  VI. Systems Development Corporation (SDC)
      2500 Colorado Avenue
      Santa Monica, CA 90406

References

(a) Williams ME, Lannom L, O'Donnell R, Barth SN. *Computer-Readable Data Bases: A Directory and Data Sourcebook*. Washington, DC. American Society for Information Science. 1979.

(b) National Library of Medicine. *Online Services Reference Manual.* Bethesda, MD. National Institutes of Health. 1980.

(c) *Directory of Online Information Resources,* 5th ed. Rockville, MD. CSG Press. 1980.

593. *Agricola*

> Producer: U.S. Department of Agricultural
> Technical Information Service
> Beltsville, MD 20705
>
> Supplier: BRS, Lockheed
>
> Broad coverage of the agricultural literature. Useful to search for toxicology of foods, food additives, plants, veterinary products, pesticides, etc.

594. *BIOSIS Previews*

> Producer: BioSciences Information Service
> 2100 Arch Street
> Philadelphia, PA 19103
>
> Supplier: BRS, Lockheed, SDC
>
> Includes biology, chemistry, agriculture, medicine and related sciences.

595. *CA Search*

> Producer: Chemical Abstracts Service
> American Chemical Society
> Ohio State University
> Columbus, OH 43210
>
> Supplier: Lockheed, SDC
>
> International coverage of chemical literature corresponding to *Chemical Abstracts*. Includes references from proceedings, technical reports, and patents as well as journals.

596. *CANCERLINE*

> Producer: International Cancer Research Data Bank Program (ICRDB)
> 9000 Rockville Pike
> Bethesda, MD 20014
>
> Supplier: NLM
>
> Data base contains records appearing in *Cancer Therapy Abstracts, Chemotherapy Abstracts, Carcinogenesis Abstracts* and is augmented by additional records. Coverage is of journal articles, technical reports, monographs, proceedings, theses, etc.

597. *CANCERPROJ*

Producer: International Cancer Research Data Bank Program (ICRDB)
9000 Rockville Pike
Bethesda, MD 20014

Supplier: NLM

Covers ongoing research projects related to cancer.

598. *CHEMDEX*

Producer: Chemical Abstracts Service
American Chemical Society
Ohio State University
Columbus, OH 43210

Supplier: SDC

Chemical dictionary on-line.

599. *CHEMLINE*

Producer: Toxicology Information Program
National Library of Medicine
8600 Rockville Pike
Bethesda, MD 20209

Supplier: NLM

On-line chemical dictionary. Contains synonyms and Chemical Abstracts names and registry numbers. Permits searching by name and formula fragments. Indicates location of files where additional data or literature citations are available. TOSCA inventory chemicals have been tagged.

600. *CHEMNAME*

Producer: Chemical Abstracts Service
American Chemical Society
Ohio State University
Columbus, OH 43210

Supplier: Lockheed

On-line chemical dictionary.

601. *ENERGYLINE*

Producer: Environmental Information Center
292 Madison Avenue
New York, NY 10017

Supplier: Lockheed, SDC

File contents include energy, resources, and environmental impacts.

602. *ENVIROLINE*

> Producer: Environmental Information Center
> 292 Madison Avenue
> New York, NY 10017
>
> Supplier: Lockheed, SDC
>
> Covers all environmental areas.

603. *Environmental Impact Statements*

> Producer: Information Resources Press
> 2100 M Street NW
> Washington, DC 20036
>
> Supplier: BRS
>
> Abstracts of EIS' as required by the National Environmental Policy Act.

604. *Excerpta Medica*

> Producer: Excerpta Medica Foundation
> Keizergracht 205
> Amsterdam
> The Netherlands
>
> Supplier: Lockheed
>
> Broad biomedical coverage of journal and selected monographic litera-
> ture. Of special interest are sections on pharmacology and toxicology,
> environmental health and pollution, adverse reactions, and cancer.

605. *IRL Life Sciences*

> Producer: Information Retrieval, Inc.
> Suite 815
> 250 West 57th Street
> New York, NY 10019
>
> Supplier: Lockheed
>
> A merged data base which contains records from a variety of biomedical
> files including *Toxicology Abstracts*.

606. *Laboratory Animal Data Bank (LADB)*

> Producer: Battelle Columbus Laboratories
> LADB Operations and Search Center
> 505 King Avenue
> Columbus, OH 43201
> (in cooperation with NLM)
>
> Supplier: Battelle Columbus Laboratories
>
> Consists of unpublished animal data concerning clinical chemistry, hus-
> bandry, hematology, environment etc. Information on location of animal
> strains is also available. Typical data elements for a given animal group

are type and schedule of lighting, feed manufacturer, crude protein and fat percentages in feed, frequency of feeding, method of feeding, etc. The *LADB* data bank may be used for breed or strain selection, for comparison of data, for establishing baseline values, to determine spontaneous disease incidence, etc.

607. *MEDLINE*

Producer: National Library of Medicine
8600 Rockville Pike
Bethesda, MD 20209

Supplier: BRS, NLM

International in scope. Broadly covers medicine and the life sciences. Searching may be done via a controlled vocabulary known as MESH (Medical Subject Headings) or via free text. Covers primarily journal articles with selected monographs.

608. *National Institute for Occupational Safety and Health Technical Information Center (NIOSHTIC)*

Producer: Clearinghouse for Occupational Safety and Health Information
Division of Technical Services
National Institute for Occupational Safety and Health
4676 Columbia Parkway
Cincinnati, OH 45226

Contact: Ted Schoenborn at above address regarding availability.

Covers all areas of occupational safety and health. Indexes journals, proceedings, meetings, symposia, plus all NIOSH documents, references cited in these documents, and translations aquired by NIOSH. Also contains selected references from CIS, the International Labour Organization's data base in Geneva. Some personal files of researchers are part of *NIOSHTIC* as well. Material dates back to the 1800's.

609. *NIH-EPA Chemical Information System (CIS)*

Producer: Interactive Sciences Corporation
CIS Project
918 16th Street, NW
Washington, DC 20006

Supplier: Interactive Sciences Corporation

Over 40 different files can be searched by this system. The files are linked by the "Structure and Nomenclature Search System" (SANSS), which is a chemical dictionary with graphics capabilities that can draw molecular structures. Among the components of CIS linked to SANSS are the "Mass Spectral Search System," "EPA's Oil and Hazardous Materials Technical Assistance Data System (OHM-TADS)," "Registry of Toxic Effects of Chemical Substances (RTECS)," "X-Ray Crystallographic Search System (CRYST)," and the "Federal Register Notices (FR) System."

610. *Pollution Abstracts*

Producer: Data Courier
620 South Fifth Street
Louisville, KY 40202

Supplier: BRS, Lockheed, SDC

Corresponds to the hard copy publication, *Pollution Abstracts.*

611. *RTECS (Registry of the Toxic Effects of Chemical Substances)*

Producer: National Institute for Occupational Safety and Health
4676 Columbia Parkway
Cincinnati, OH 45226

Supplier: Interactive Sciences Corporation, NLM

The on-line equivalent of NIOSH's hard copy, annually compiled *RTECS.* This factual data bank contains information on over 35,000 substances. Searchable by prime name, synonyms, class of compounds, Chemical Abstracts registry number, etc. Provides toxicity data including aquatic toxicity.

612. *SCISEARCH*

Producer: Institute for Scientific Information
3501 Market Street
University City Science Center
Philadelphia, PA 19104

Supplier: BRS, Lockheed

Multidisciplinary scientific file. Unique feature allows searching by cited references.

613. *Toxicology Data Bank (TDB)*

Producer: Toxicology Information Program
National Library of Medicine
8600 Rockville Pike
Bethesda, MD 20209

Supplier: NLM

This on-line factual data bank contains information on chemical substances from over 60 peer reviewed monographs. Contains approximately 25,000 records (completed and in process). Information on nomenclature, threshold limit values, pharmacology/toxicology, environment, manufacture, and chemical/physical constants is provided.

614. *TOXLINE*

Producer: Toxicology Information Program
National Library of Medicine
8600 Rockville Pike
Bethesda, MD 20209

Supplier: NLM

A major file for bibliographic information (primarily periodical literature) on chemicals, drugs, toxicology, pharmacology. The database is a merger of the following subfiles: 1. Chemical-Biological Activities 2. Toxicity Bibliography 3. Abstracts on the Health Effects of Environmental Pollutants 4. International Pharmaceutical Abstracts 5. Pesticides Abstracts 6. Environmental Mutagen Information Center file 7. TERA (a teratology file) 8. A pesticides file compiled by WJ Hayes, JR 9. the Toxicology/Epidemiology Research Projects Directory. TOXBACK indexes literature generally prior to 1974. TOXLINE and TOXBACK combined contain about 1 million records. Generally a free text data base.

615. *TSCA*

Producer: US Environmental Protection Agency
Office of Pesticides and Toxic Substances
Division of Chemical Information
401 M Street SW
Washington, DC 20460

Supplier: Lockheed

Covers the list of commercial chemicals in the initial inventory of the Toxic Substances Control Act.

615a. *UPGRADE*

Producer: Sigma Data Computing Corp.
2021 K Street
Suite 207
Washington, DC 20006

Supplier: Sigma Data Computing Corp.

UPGRADE (User-Prompted Graphic Data Evaluation) system produces elegant statistical and graphic displays, including maps, derived from numeric data bases. Available data bases include EPA's SAROAD (air quality), STORET (water quality), the National Center for Health Statistics data base on mortality and health statistics, plus files from the Department of Energy, the US Census Bureau, the Geological Survey, and assorted state agencies. Statistics on topics such as cancer mortality can be plotted and shown as densities on a map.

Chapter 12

Directories

Among the directories listed have been mostly those of organizations. Two of the directories, the *Encyclopedia of Associations* and the *United States Government Manual* cover groups with a variety of interests other than toxicology, but they have been selected because they are excellent general tools. Virtually every organization has a membership directory, listing individual names. These have not been listed. Unfortunately, there does not exist one directory to satisfy all the toxicologist's needs. The National Referral Center's *Directory of Information Resources in the United States: General Toxicology* comes closest but it needs intensive updating and is too old to be of much practical value.

For other publications which may serve the purposes of directories, see the *Annual Reports* section of this guide.

616. Colle J, ed. *Federal activities in toxic substances*. Washington, DC. Office of Pesticides and Toxic Substances, US Environmental Protection Agency. 1980. (EPA-560/13-80-015)

> Part of the *Toxics Integration Information Series*. Lists information on CPSC, CEQ, DOA, DHHS, DOL, DOT, EPA, and the National Toxicology Program. Organizational charts, divisions concerned with toxics, and phone numbers are provided, as well as substantial text indicating what the agency's activities are.

616a. Colle J, Slike KA, compilers. *Directory of Federal Coordinating Groups for Toxic Substances,* 2nd ed. Washington, DC. United States Environmental Protection Agency, Office of Toxic Substances. 1980.

> Part of the *Toxics Integration Information Series* of EPA, this directory lists coordinative groups in toxicology, member agencies with ad-

dresses, names, and phone numbers. A personnel index allows for location of group affiliation. The first edition of this directory also had agency indexes, which permitted determination of which coordinative groups a given agency belonged to. This feature has been inexplicably deleted from the 2nd edition.

617. *Contact:Toxics: A guide to specialists on toxic substances.* New York. World Environment Center. 1980.

Designed *only* for the use of the news media and professionals, this unique directory lists about 1000 specialists in toxics, from throughout the country. Individuals chosen from various sectors (e.g., government, academia, etc.). Indexed by chemicals, technologies, environmental issues. Addresses, phone numbers, brief biographical sketches and specialties are listed. Includes a table of priority pollutants, a chronology of major acts, a technical glossary and a list of acronyms.

618. *Directory of Academic Programs in Occupational Safety and Health.* Cincinatti, OH. United States Department of Health, Education, and Welfare, Public Health Service, Center for Disease Control, National Institute of Occupational Safety and Health, Division of Training and Manpower Development. 1979.

Lists associate, certificate, baccalaureate, and advanced degree programs in occupational safety and health, industrial hygiene, occupational health nursing, and occupational medicine. Among the schools are NIOSH's twelve Educational Resource Centers, which participate in a special grants program.

619. *Directory of Government Agencies Safeguarding Consumer and Environment.* Alexandria, VA. Serina Press. 1978.

Lists federal and state agencies in areas such as food and drugs, meat and poultry inspection, poison control, consumer product safety, air pollution, water pollution, noise abatement, etc.

620. *Directory of Poison Control Centers.* In *Bulletin—National Clearinghouse for Poison Control Centers.* 24(8), Aug 1980.

Compiled from information received from poison control centers and state health departments. Divided geographically by state and includes addresses, phone numbers, and state coordinators. Published each August in the *Bulletin.*

621. *Directory of Pollution Control Officials.* In *The Environment Index 79.* New York. Environment Information Center. 1979.

Consists of listings of EPA regional offices, regional commissions on pollution control, US Army Corps of Engineers Divisons and Districts, and state control offices in air pollution, pesticides, radiation, solid waste, and water pollution.

622. Emerson PR, McFadden JE, compilers. *Directory of Federal Interagency Groups Concerned with Environmental Health,* 2nd ed. Gaithersburg, MD. GEOMET. 1980

Prepared by the Task Force on Environmental Cancer and Heart and Lung Disease. Information listed includes membership, charter by which group was created, activities, publications and products, schedules of meetings, duration of the committee, and work groups. Agency and individual representative indexes. Updated biannually in April and October.

623. *Encyclopedia of Associations.* Detroit. Gale Research. 1961–

"Comprehensive source of detailed information concerning nonprofit American membership organizations of national scope. In it can be found the location, size, objectives, and many other essential aspects of several thousand trade associations, professional societies, labor unions, fraternal and patriotic organizations, and other types of groups consisting of voluntary members." In addition *selected* for-profit groups, nonmembership groups, foreign, international, local, regional, and citizen action groups are included.

624. Gough BE. *World Environment Directory,* 4th ed. Silver Spring, MD. Business Publishers. 1980.

Part I of this giant directory is devoted to US companies, agencies, and organizations. Among the many categories into which this part is divided are product manufacturers (for air, water, noise control pollution equipment, etc.), government agencies, attorneys specializing in the environment, state agencies, public interest groups, corporate environmental officials, etc. Part II is devoted to foreign organizations.

625. *Mutagenicity Testing Laboratories in the U.S.* Michael D. Shelby. Office of the Associate Director for Genetics. National Institute of Environmental Health Sciences. Research Triangle Park, NC 27709. April 1980.

Includes commercial, nonprofit, and university labs that routinely offer their testing services. For each lab, there is an address, phone number, and contact person plus a list of all the tests they engage in (both available assay systems and those under development). Listed both alphabetically by lab name and geographically by state. Includes an index by the assay system used (e.g., can be used to find list of labs doing sister-chromatid exchange). A very handy directory which will be hopefully kept up to date.

626. National Referral Center for Science and Technology. *A Directory of Information Resources in the United States: General Toxicology.* Washington, DC. Library of Congress. 1969.

A directory of organizations (governmental, industrial, and academic) concerned with toxicology. Detailed subject and geographic indexes. List of periodicals and poison control centers. Unfortunately, this title is woefully outdated but an expanded version is being contemplated.

627. Thibeau CE, ed. *NFEC Directory of Environmental Information Sources.* Boston. National Foundation for Environmental Control. 1972.

Covers organizations active in environmental issues. Includes lists of abstracts, bibliographies, conferences, serials, books, film. Could use updating.

628. *United States Government Manual.* Washington, DC. General Services Administration, National Archives and Records Service, Office of the Federal Register. 1973/74–

The official handbook of the US Federal Government, published annually. Information on agencies of the legislative, judicial, and executive branches of the government. Independent establishments, government corporations, quasi-official agencies, and selected multilateral and bilateral organizations are listed. Organizational charts for selected agencies and listing of higher level administrators for most agencies provided.

629. *US Directory of Environmental Sources,* 2nd ed. Washington, D.C. U.S. International Environmental Referral Center. 1977. [NTIS #—PB 274 110]

Lists organizations registered with the U.S. National Focal Point of the United Nations Environment Program's International Referral System. Information provided includes organization sponsorship, activities, functions, publications and a brief description. Indexed by the International Referral System's subject thesaurus (known as ''subject attributes'').

PART II

ORGANIZATIONS

The organizations have been divided into three areas—governmental, non-governmental, and federal coordinative. Governmental organizations are limited to the United States federal government and may include full fledged agencies and departments as well as bureaus or divisions within the larger group if they are sufficiently important to warrant inclusion within this list. Governmental organizations tend to be notoriously unwieldy and although their numerous subdivisons may be organizationally independent on paper, they are rarely mutually exclusive in reality. Agencies as total entities also have overlapping concerns and trying to track down all the governmental activity in hazards associated with synthetic fuels, say, can be a definite chore. Still, the United States government is a primary source for recent information in toxicology, from both the scientific and regulatory viewpoints. On another level, although not included in this bibliography, is the work being performed by state, local, and regional agencies, planning boards, etc. concerned with the environment, toxic substances, and hazardous wastes.

Nongovernmental organizations include independent associations, professional groups, accrediting and certifying boards, and private research institutes. Industrial firms have not been included. Haskell Labs (Dupont) and Monsanto are just two examples of private industrial laboratories that are doing extensive and outstanding work in toxicity testing. Because of TOSCA and the responsibility of industry to generate and report vast amounts of quality-controlled toxicity data, private industry will become an increasingly valuable resource for toxicological information.

Coordinative groups consist of two or more independent groups that have joined forces to address particular issues that affect them all. The intention is to avoid duplication of effort, control the flow of information, keep members abreast of each other's developments, and increase overall efficiency. Although the coordinative groups play a valuable role in pooling efforts and reducing redundancy, they have proliferated to such an extent that the questions of duplication among even these groups has arisen and soon it may be necessary to have a coordinative group to coordinate the coordinative groups. This is a question that deserves further investigation.

A group that is all but invisible in this organizational morass is that of contractors. Because of budgetary constraints, need for greater expertise in certain projects, and other reasons, organizations, especially the federal government, are increasingly relying on ''contracting out'' work. Many of the reports finally issued by government agencies have really been prepared by contractors. This information may or may not be apparent by examining the final document of a study. A list of contractors has been omitted, although it would be informative to have such a list, see who the contractors are, what proportion of toxicology spending is going to contractors, and what agencies are making the heaviest use of them.

Names and telephone numbers have generally not been included because they are too subject to change. Exceptions to this are individual names and organizational affiliations that *have* been included for coordinative groups because they are not usually stationed (as a group) at one physical location. Of course, even the organizational names listed are subject to change. What was long known as the Office of Toxic Substances is currently called the Office of Pesticides and Toxic Substances. Shifts in organizational structure and responsibility, too, are routine occurences. The usual run-around in locating the proper individual in an organization is unavoidable. On one occasion I was transferred seven times between two cities trying to find information about a publication issued by a major governmental agency.

With the 1980 change of administration in Washington and the emphasis on budget cutting and regulatory reform, it is not likely that the early 1980s will see changes in the structure and function of the federal organizations in this chapter as well as alterations in the regulations applicable to the laws in the following chapter. It appears possible that the focus of regulatory concerns will be shifted from the federal to the state level.

Chapter 13

Governmental Organizations

630. *Bureau of Radiological Health (BRH)*
12720 Twinbrook Parkway, Rockville, MD 20857

Responsible for protecting public health by reducing unnecessary exposure to both ionizing and nonionizing radiation, with major emphasis on electronic product radiation control. The Bureau is assigned to the FDA. Its responsibilities in environmental radiation were transferred to the EPA in 1970.

631. *Centers for Disease Control (CDC)*
1600 Clifton Road, N.E., Atlanta, GA 30333

Charged with protecting the public health of the nation by providing leadership and direction in the prevention and control of diseases and other preventable conditions. NIOSH and the Bureau of Epidemiology are two of CDC's eight operating components.

632. *Chemical Hazard Response Information System (CHRIS)*
U.S. Coast Guard, 400 Seventh St, S.W., Washington, DC 20590

CHRIS provides timely information essential for proper decisionmaking by Coast Guard personnel and others during emergencies involving the water transport of hazardous chemicals. Another purpose is the compilation of basic nonemergency-related information to support the Coast Guard in its efforts to achieve improved levels of safety in the bulk shipment of hazardous chemicals.

633. *Chemical Monograph Referral Center (CHEMRIC)*
Consumer Product Safety Commission, 5401 Westbard Avenue Room 700, Bethesda, MD 20207

CHEMRIC's mission is to receive and disseminate information on contemplated, planned, in-progress, and completed monographs and criteria documents on chemical compounds or families of compounds, with special emphasis on toxicological properties of chemicals, among federal health-related agencies and other organizations. The intent is to prevent the unknowing duplication of monographs on the same compound.

634. *Consumer Product Safety Commission (CPSC)*
1111 Eighteenth Street NW, Washington, DC 20207

Purpose is to protect the public against unreasonable risks of injury from consumer products; to assist consumers to evaluate the comparative safety of consumer products and minimize conflicting state and local regulations; and to promote research and investigation into the causes and prevention of product-related deaths, illnesses, and injuries.

635. *Council on Environmental Quality (CEQ)*
722 Jackson Place N.W., Washington, D.C. 20006

Established by the National Environmental Policy Act of 1969 to formulate and recommend national policies to promote the quality of the environment. The Toxic Substances Strategy Committee (TSSC) chaired by CEQ was formed to develop an interagency program to eliminate overlaps and fill gaps in collection of data on toxic chemicals and to coordinate federal research and regulatory activities affecting them.

636. *Department of Agriculture (USDA)*
Fourteenth Street and Independence Avenue S.W., Washington, D.C. 20250

The Food Safety and Quality Service (FSQS) is a quality control division, which insures that foods are safe and nutritious and accurately labeled. USDA also encourages safe use of pesticides and is active in environmental conservation programs.

637. *Department of Energy (DOE)*
1000 Independence Avenue S.W., Washington, D.C. 20545

DOE's environment program is responsible for ensuring that the implementation of all departmental programs is consistent with environmental and safety laws, regulations, and policies. Also conducted are environmental and health-related research and development programs, such as studies of energy-related pollutants and their effects on biological systems.

638. *Department of Transportation (DOT)*
400 Seventh St S.W., Washington, DC 20590

The Materials Transportation Bureau was formed to coordinate DOT's increasing overall responsibilities concerning hazardous materials transportation and pipeline safety. The US Coast Guard is also a component of DOT and is responsible for shipment of toxic substances.

639. *Environmental Mutagen Information Center (EMIC)*
Oak Ridge National Laboratory, Oak Ridge, Tennessee 37830

Collects and disseminates chemical mutagenic information. The EMIC data base is one of the TOXLINE subfiles. Questions that cannot be answered on-line may be directed to the center. The center also maintains an Agent Registry file of information on all the chemical agents in the EMIC file.

640. *Environmental Teratogen Information Center (ETIC)*
Oak Ridge National Laboratory, Oak Ridge, Tennessee 37830

This center follows concepts similar to EMIC. Literature containing data reporting on the testing of chemical, physical, and biological agents for teratogenic activity in warm-blooded animals is being located and collected. Particular attention is given to papers that implicate agents in the production of congenital defects in man.

641. *Environmental Protection Agency (EPA)*
401 M Street S.W., Washington, DC 20460

EPA's mission is to control and abate pollution in the areas of air, water, solid waste, noise, radiation, and toxic substances. EPA's mandate is to mount an integrated, coordinated attack on environmental pollution in cooperation with state and local governments. There are programs in air and waste management, water and hazardous materials, and toxic substances. The Office of Pesticides and Toxic Substances coordinates activities under the Toxic Substances Control Act with other agencies for the assessment and control of toxic substances.

642. *Food and Drug Administration (FDA)*
5600 Fishers Lane, Rockville, MD 20857

FDA activities are directed toward protecting the health of the nation against impure and unsafe foods, drugs, and cosmetics, and other potential hazards. Among its branches are: Bureau of Drugs, Bureau of Biologics, Bureau of Foods, Bureau of Radiological Health, Bureau of Veterinary Medicine, Bureau of Medical Devices, and the National Center for Toxicological Research.

643. *Information Response to Chemical Crises (IRCC) Project*
Toxicology Information Response Center
Oak Ridge National Laboratory, Oak Ridge, TN 37830

Sponsored by the DHHS CCER, the Department of Agriculture, EPA,
NIEHS, and NOAA, this project is designed to offer rapid access to
information/literature on given chemicals or topics of a crises nature.
Noncrises topics shall be nominated and will also result in bibliographies
and literature searches. This service is only available to project member
Federal organizations.

644. *National Cancer Institute (NCI)*
9000 Rockville Pike, Bethesda, MD 20014

Toxicology research at NCI includes the identification of populations at
increased cancer risk resulting from exposures to chemicals; investigations on the effects and biological fate of carcinogens and structurally
similar compounds; development of new methods for detecting chemical
carcinogens; bioassay studies to identify and evaluate environmental
carcinogens; studies on the pharmacological and other biological properties of potential cancer chemotherapeutic agents; and clinical studies to
characterize the toxicity of cancer chemotherapeutic agents.

645. *National Center for Toxicological Research (NCTR)*
Jefferson, AR 72079

Toxicological research and development studies to evaluate effects of
food additives, drugs, veterinary products, and environmental pollutants, including protocols for carcinogencity, teratogenicity, mutagenicity, histopathology, and general clinical pathology. NCTR is a component of FDA.

646. *National Clearinghouse of Poison Control Centers (NCPCC)*
Poison Control Division, Bureau of Drugs
5401 Westbard Avenue, Bethesda, MD 20016

Assists poison control centers in this country. Collects data on poisons
and hazardous products that is indexed on cards. Encourages
epidemiologic research. Publishes a monthly bulletin.

647. *National Council on Radiation Protection and Measurements*
7910 Woodmont Avenue, Suite 1016, Bethesda, MD 20014

Composed of scientific experts who make recommendations on radiation
protection and promote cooperation among organizations concerned with
radiation problems. The Council cooperates with the International
Commission on Radiological Protection.

648. *National Library of Medicine (NLM)*
8600 Rockville Pike, Bethesda, MD 20209

NLM, the largest medical library in the world, collects extensively in health related aspects of toxicology. NLM produced or maintained data bases include MEDLINE, TOXLINE, TDB, RTECS, LADB. The Specialized Information Services (SIS) division is heavily involved in toxicology information activities.

649. *National Electronic Injury Surveillance System (NEISS)*
Consumer Product Safety Commission
1111 Eighteenth Street N.W., Washington, DC 20207

Operated by the US Consumer Product Safety Commission. Through a network of over 100 hospitals, data is transmitted on product related injuries. Hazard patterns are analyzed.

650. *National Institute of Environmental Health Sciences (NIEHS)*
PO Box 12233, Research Triangle Park, NC 27709

The principal Federal agency for the support of research and the training of research manpower, in the area of the effects of chemical, physical, and biological environmental agents on human health. Its primary mission is to conduct and support biomedical research which will identify, characterize, and prevent the adverse effects of environmental agents on human health. Most of NIEHS' research and development activities can be divided between basic toxicology research and toxicology method development and validation.

651. *National Institute for Occupational Safety and Health (NIOSH)*
5600 Fishers Lane, Rockville, MD 20857

Areas of interest include: occupational health, industrial hygiene, toxicology and hazards of industrial materials and conditions; chemical, engineering, nursing, medicinal, and physiological aspects of occupational health hazards, prevention and treatment of injurious effects on health, poisonous gases, vapors, mist, and dust, radiation, heat and humidity, noise, effects of pesticides.

652. *National Oceanic and Atmospheric Administration (NOAA)*
6010 Executive Boulevard, Rockville, MD 20852

NOAA explores and charts the global ocean and its resources. It predicts conditions in the atmosphere and issues warnings against natural disasters. NOAA has programs to protect marine mammals and conserve marine resources. It conducts research on alternatives to ocean dumping. It operates a national environmental satellite system and collects and disseminates worldwide environmental data.

653. *Nuclear Regulatory Commission (NRC)*
1717 H Street N.W., Washington, DC 20555

Licenses and regulates the uses of nuclear energy to protect the public health and safety and the environment. Among the items under its control are nuclear reactors and other nuclear facilities, and the handling and disposal of nuclear materials.

654. *Occupational Safety and Health Administration (OSHA)*
200 Constitution Avenue, N.W., Washington, DC 20210

Develops and promulgates occupational safety and health standards; develops and issues regulations; conducts investigations and inspections to determine the status of safety and health standards and regulations; and issues citations and proposes penalties for noncompliance with safety and health standards and regulations.

655. *Toxicology Information Center*
National Academy of Sciences
2600 Virginia Avenue, Washington, DC 20418

The center is part of NAS' Committee on Toxicology and serves primarily a limited number of government agencies in providing information. Over 80 journals are scanned for toxicology literature and a card file is maintained by chemical. Experts in toxicology serve on the committee on a rotational basis and are responsible for preparation of reports. The group addresses policy matters and reviews research protocols. The center concentrates on industrial-environmental chemicals and food additives.

656. *Toxicology Information Program (TIP)*
Division of Specialized Information Services
National Library of Medicine
8600 Rockville Pike, Bethesda, MD 20209

General objectives are to create computer-based toxicology data banks from the scientific literature and from the files of collaborating industrial academic, and governmental agencies and to establish toxicology information services for the scientific community.

657. *Toxicology Information Response Center (TIRC)*
P.O. Box X, Building 2024, Room 53, Oak Ridge, TN 37830

TIRC provides extensive toxicology information and reference services to the scientific, administrative, and public communities on individual chemicals, chemical classes, and a wide variety of toxicology-related topics.

Chapter 14

Nongovernmental Organizations

658. *American Academy of Clinical Toxicology*
Walter Decker, Secretary-Treasurer
Department of Pharmacology and Toxicology
University of Texas Medical Branch, Galveston, TX 77550

The Academy is composed of both physicians and nonphysicians. The Academy holds meetings, sponsors continuing education, and supports any other initiatives in clinical toxicology.

659. *American Academy of Forensic Sciences*
11400 Rockville Pike, Rockville, MD 20852

Interested in improving research into and study of standards in the fields of forensic sciences.

660. *American Association of Poison Control Centers*
c/o William O. Robertson, MD
Children's Orthopedic Hospital
P.O. Box C-5371, Seattle, WA 98105

Procures information on the ingredients and potential acute toxicity of substances that may cause accidental poisonings and establishes standard for poison information and control centers.

661. *American Board of Medical Toxicology*
Dr. Frederick H. Lovejoy, Jr. Chairman
Harvard Medical School/Children's Hospital Medical Center
300 Longwood Avenue, Boston, MA 02115

The board establishes standards for the training and qualifications of physicians specializing in clinical toxicology. Certification is available by examination.

662. *American Chemical Society (ACS)*
1155 16th Street, N.W., Washington, DC 20036

Professional association of chemists and chemical engineers. Educational and career services. Numerous committees and divisions. Publishes some two dozen journals. Some divisions of interest to toxicologists are Agriculture and Food, Chemical Health and Safety, Environmental, and Pesticide.

663. *American College of Toxicology*
c/o Dr. Richard E. Kouri
Microbiological Associates
5221 River Road, Bethesda, MD 20016

One of the newer professional organizations, ACT promotes various aspects of the field of toxicology. Its first annual meeting was held in 1979.

664. *American College of Veterinary Toxicologists*
W. Eugene Lloyd, President
College of Veterinary Medicine
Iowa State University, Ames, Iowa 50011

Encourages progress in veterinary toxicology. Sponsors workshops, symposia.

665. *American Industrial Hygiene Association*
475 Wolf Ledges Parkway, Akron, OH 44311

Interest in industrial hygiene, air pollution, aerosols, analytical chemistry, biochemical assays, contaminant control, noise, radiation, toxicology. Publishes *American Industrial Hygiene Association Journal*.

666. *Chemical Industry Institute of Toxicology (CIIT)*
P.O. Box 12137, Research Triangle Park, NC 27709

Studies potential toxic hazards of commodity chemicals in relation to the manufacture, handling, use, and ultimate disposal of such chemicals. Answers inquiries on selected commodity chemicals. Provides advisory services and information on research in progress. CIIT is an association of chemical companies. CIIT has departments of toxicology, pathology, biochemical toxicology, genetic toxicology, and epidemiology. Fellowship appointments are available for postgraduate research and training.

667. *Chemical Manufacturers Association (CMA)*
      1825 Connecticut Avenue N.W., Washington, DC 20009

The trade association serving as the spokesman for the chemical industry. Among CMA's many committees are ones on chemical regulations,
environmental management, and occupational safety and health. Publishes literature for both the general public and professionals engaged in
the chemical industry. One of CMA's services is the "Chemical Transportation Emergency Center" (CHEMTREC), which provides information and aid in emergencies involving hazardous materials.

668. *Conservation Foundation*
      1717 Massachusetts Avenue NW, Washington, DC 20036

A research and communication organization promoting conservation of
the environment. A program in pollution control and toxic substances
initiates projects to assist in implementing environmental laws regarding
drinking water, and pesticides. This program's publications list includes
many legal documents, petitions, complaints, motions, testimony, etc.
that they have issued to assorted groups.

669. *Cosmetic, Toiletry, and Fragrance Association (CTFA)*
      1133 15th Street, N.W., Washington, DC 20005

Consists of manufacturers and distributors of cosmetics and related
products. Research in safety testing. Publishes a Legislative Bulletin, a
Trademark Bulletin, and a Cosmetic Journal

670. *Environmental Defense Fund (EDF)*
      475 Park Avenue South, New York, NY 10016

An organization spearheaded by teams of lawyers and scientists dedi-
cated to protecting the environment. The Toxic Chemicals Program has
been very active and has brought suits against EPA over asbestos, drinking water, and pesticides. This program's publications list includes many
legal documents, petitions, complaints, motions, testimony, etc. that
they have issued to assorted groups.

671. *Environmental Information Center (EIC) Inc.*
      292 Madison Avenue, New York, NY 10017

A major clearinghouse for environmental and energy information. Maintains numerous data banks and produces reference products such as
Environment Abstracts. Information services, such as document retrieval
and literature searching, are available.

672. *Environmental Law Institute*
      1346 Connecticut Avenue NW, Suite 620, Washington, DC 20036

A research, information, and educational organization in environmental law. Sponsors classes and conferences. Maintains a 5000 volume library. Publishes the monthly *Environmental Law Reporters*. The Institute has been designated a clearinghouse for collection of Environmental Impact Statements and has a nearly complete collection.

673. *Institute of Clinical Toxicology*
5410 LaBranch, Houston, TX 77006

A nonprofit teaching, service, and research organization established to further the development of clinical toxicology as a specialty concerned with diseases caused by toxic substances.

674. *International Society on Toxinology*
Box 323, 100 North State Street, Los Angeles, CA 90033

Areas of interest include pharmacology, biochemistry, and immunology of animal venoms; nature of venom apparatus and envenomations; food intoxications cause by naturally occuring plant and animal toxins. Publishes the journal *Toxicon*.

675. *National Council on Radiation Protection and Measurements*
7910 Woodmont Ave. Suite 1016, Washington, DC 20014

Members cooperate in fostering radiation protection. Publishes numerous reports. Among its committees are Biological Aspects of Radiation Protection Criteria and Biological Effects and Exposure Criteria for Radiofrequency Electromagnetic Radiation.

676. *National Poison Center Network (NPCN)*
Children's Hospital of Pittsburgh
125 DeSoto Street, Pittsburgh, PA 15213

NPCN attempts to provide standardized poison information to physicians and the public through its national network of regional and satellite centers. Each of these centers is staffed by a poison information specialist backed up by a physician, who are on duty around the clock. Each center may communicate with the National Headquarters and transmit information by telecopies. The centers are active in continuing education programs. NPCN publishes a bulletin, a membership directory, and a sourcebook.

677. *Pharmaceutical Manufacturers Association (PMA)*
1155 15th Street, Washington, DC 20005

Represents most of the drug industry in this country. Consists of biological, medical, quality control, research development, and other sections.

678. *Society of Toxicology (SOT)*
475 Wolf Ledge Parkway, Akron, OH 44311

Interested in all aspects of toxicology. SOT is the primary professional group for toxicologists. It publishes the journal *Toxicology and Applied Pharmacology*. Annual meeting.

679. *Toxicology Laboratory Accreditation Board*
600 New Hampshire Avenue, NW, Suite 720, Washington, DC 20037

Promotes high standards in toxicology by accrediting competent labs. Accreditation is based on application information and an on site visit.

Chapter 15

Federal Coordinative Groups

680. *Chemical Substances Information Network (CSIN)*
Chairman, Dr. Henry H. Kissman
Chemical Substances Information Network
National Library of Medicine
8600 Rockville Pike, Bethesda, MD 20209

This is a subcommittee of the *Interagency Toxic Substances Data Committee*. It is charged with designing, implementing, and maintaining efficient and effective systems for the storage, retrieval, and analysis of data on the effects of chemical substances on biological systems and the environment. The system will link existing and newly developed toxicology and chemical files into a network. A chemical data base directory will lead the user to various files. The network is intended to satisfy the information gathering requirements of TOSCA and to also be of value to researchers, government, academia, and concerned citizen groups.

681. *DHHS Committee to Coordinate Environmental and Related Programs (CCERP)*
Executive Secretary, Dr. Raymond Shapiro
DHHS Committee to Coordinate Environmental and Related Programs
P.O. Box 12233, Research Triangle Park, NC 27709

A multiagency group designed to provide a medium to assure the exchange of information on environmental health, toxicology, and related programs, to coordinate the programs, and to promote resource-sharing. The following standing committees have been established: Subcommittee on Environmental Mutagenesis, Subcommittee on Laboratory Chemical Carcinogen Safety Standards, Toxicology Information Subcommittee, Subcommittee to Coordinate Polybrominated Biphenyls within the Public Health Service, and the Subcommittee to Coordinate Asbestos/ ''Asbestiform'' Research within the Public Health Service.

682. *Federal Interagency Committee on the Health and Environmental Effects of Energy Technologies*
Executive Secretariat, Dr. Richard Brown
Mitre Corporation
1820 Dolly Madison Boulevard
Mail Stop W308, McLean, VA 22101

Consisting of NIEHS, NIOSH, DOE, and EPA, this committee is examining health and environmental problems associated with energy technologies. The committee sponsors workshops and establishes working groups.

683. *Federal Interagency Noise Research Coordination Panel*
Jack Shampan
Environmental Protection Agency
ONAC (ANR 471)
Washington, DC 20460

The panel reviews activities on noise effects, identifies and prioritizes research needs, and generally coordinates Federal noise effects research.

684. *Gene-Tox Steering Committee*
Chairman, Dr. Angela Auletta
Office of Pesticides and Toxic Substances
Health Review Division
Environmental Protection Agency
TS-792
401 M Street, SW, Washington, DC 20460

Coordinates evaluation of bioassays (*in vivo* and *in vitro*) in use for mutagenesis.

685. *Interagency Collaborative Group on Environmental Carcinogensis (ICGEC)*
Chairman, Dr. H. F. Kraybill
Scientific Coordinator for Environmental Cancer
Division of Cancer Cause and Prevention
National Cancer Institute
7910 Woodmont Avenue, Landow Building, Room 3C37, Bethesda, MD 20205

A forum for information exchange among Federal agencies concerned with environmental health and environmental carcinogensis. Also provides NCI with a resource for program development using monitoring systems and resources of other agencies to delineate levels of environmental exposure to carcinogens in man's media (e.g., air, water, workplace).

686. *Interagency Radiation Research Committee (IRRC)*
Dr. Joseph G. Perpich
Associate Director for Program Planning and Evaluation
9000 Rockville Pike
Building 1, Room 137, Bethesda, MA 20205

Established in June 1980. Chartered by DHHS Secretary Harris pursuant to a presidential mandate, this committee is the successor to the *Committee on Federal Research into the Biological Effects of Ionizing Radiation*. It is responsible for preparing an agenda for federal research into the biological effects of ionizing radiation and determining future research strategies. Member agencies are USDA, Department of Commerce, Department of Defense, DOE, DHHS (Office of the General Counsel, CDC, NIOSH, FDA, NIH), Department of Labor, DOT, CPSC, EPA, FEMA, NASA, NSF, NRC, and the Veterans Administration.

687. *Interagency Regulatory Liason Group (IRLG)*
Dr. Allen H. Heim
Scientific Coordinator for Interagency Affairs (HF-8)
Food and Drug Administration
5600 Fishers Lane, Rockville, MD 20857

The purpose of this agency is to increase coopration between the member agencies, make the most efficient use of resources, achieve consistent regulatory policy, and improve the protection of the public health and environment. The members are FDA, EPA, OSHA, CPSC, and the Food Safety and Quality Service of the Department of Agriculture. Eight work groups have been developed in compliance and enforcement, education and communications, epidemiology, information exchange, regulatory development, risk assessment, testing standards and guidelines, and research planning.

688. *Interagency Toxic Substances Data Committee (ITSDC)*
Co-Chairperson, Carroll Leslie Bastian
Council on Environmental Quality
722 Jackson Place N.W., Washington, DC 20006

Jointly established and co-chaired by the Environmental Protection Agency and the Council on Environmental Quality in accordance with statutory responsibilities under the Toxic Substances Control Act. The committee coordinates the planning and activities concerning chemical data and information projects of the major Federal producers and users of chemical data. It also studies ways to improve the collection, analysis, and exchange of data among Federal agencies and other user groups. Two important subcommittees are the *Chemical Substances Information Network (CSIN)* and the *Toxicology Information Subcommittee (TIS)*.

689. *National Response Team*
Chairman, Mr. Kenneth E. Biglane
Environmental Protection Agency
Oil and Special Materials Control Division
WH 548
401 M Street S.W., Washington, DC 20460

The national body for planning and preparedness for emergencies involving releases to the environment. Some of the primary agencies involved are the Department of Commerce, the US Geological Survey, the National Oceanic and Atmospheric Administration, and the US Coast Guard.

690. *National Toxicology Program (NTP)*
Dr. John A. Moore
Deputy Director, National Toxicology Program Sciences
National Institute of Environmental Health Sciences
P.O. Box 12233, Research Triangle Park, NC 27709

The broad goal of this program is to strengthen DHEW's activities in the testing of chemicals of public health concern, as well as in the development and validation of new and better integrated test methods. Specific goals of the program are 1. to broaden toxicological characterization of those chemicals being tested; 2. to increase the rate of chemical testing, within the limits of available resources; 3. to develop and begin to validate a series of protocols more appropriate for regulatory needs. An informative annual plan is issued. NTP is composed of FDA, NCI, CDC/NIOSH, and NIEHS.

691. *The Regulatory Council*
Peter J. Petkas
Director
United States Regulatory Council
Washington, DC 20503

Announced by President Carter in 1978 as part of his Regulatory Reform Program, this council's purpose is to improve the coordination of Federal regulatory activities and expand efforts to manage the regulatory process more effectively. The Council is composed of 16 Executive Departments and Agencies and 19 Independent Regulatory Agencies. The Council publishes the *Calendar of Federal Regulations* (see *Fugitive Literature*) every 6 months in the Federal Register. Although environmental health is a primary concern of the council, its activities deal with other areas as well.

692. *Task Force on Environmental Cancer and Heart and Lung Disease*
Contact: Dr. George R. Simon
Science Review Administrator
Environmental Protection Agency
401 M Street, SW, Washington, DC 20460

Participating agencies are various components of DHHS and EPA. The task force's primary objective is to recommend a comprehensive research program in uncovering the connection between the environment and heart and lung disease, and to develop a strategy to combat such environmentally induced diseases.

693. *Toxic Substances Strategy Committee (TSSC)*
Executive Secretary, Dr. Bob Nicholas
Senior Staff Member
Council on Environmental Quality
722 Jackson Place, NW, Washington, DC 20006

Chaired by the CEQ, this committee was instructed to develop an interagency agenda to eliminate duplication and fill gaps in the collection of toxic chemical data, and to coordinate research and regulatory activities of the Federal government in this area. TSSC has recently issued its report to the President (see *Toxic Chemicals and Public Protection* under *Monographs*).

694. *TSCA Interagency Testing Committee*
Dr. James M. Sontag
Assistant to the Director
Division of Cancer Cause and Prevention
National Cancer Institute
Building 31, Room 3A16, Bethesda, MD 20205

The committee identifies and recommends to the Administrator of EPA those chemical substances and mixtures that should be tested to determine their hazards to the health of humans and the environment. A screening procedure identifies substances and categories of substances that require priority testing.

PART III

LEGISLATION AND REGULATIONS

Chapter 16

Legislation and Regulations

There is a vast amount of toxic substance legislation and regulations in existence. Conflicting authorities for administration of various areas of concern is not unusual. Many federal, state, and local agencies are involved in hazardous substance control, as well. The names of the laws in this section are drawn from the 1976 U.S. Code's "Popular Names and Tables" index. Along with each law is its PL or Stat. number and the year it was enacted. Laws are compiled annually in the *US Statutes at Large* (a) and codified in the *US Code* (b). The *Federal Register* (c) is issued daily and provides rules and regulations as well as notices, proposed rules, and presidential proclamations. Annually, the regulations are codified in the *Code of Federal Regulations* (CFR) (d).

Of the 50 titles that comprise the *US Code,* the following contain especially useful toxicologically related law:

- 7. Agriculture
- 15. Commerce and Trade
- 16. Conservation
- 21. Food and Drugs
- 27. Intoxicating Liquors
- 39. Mineral Lands and Mining
- 42. Public Health and Welfare
- 46. Shipping
- 49. Transportation

Following are suggestions for searching the US Codes General Index (starred terms are particularly helpful):

Air Pollution Prevention and Control
Atomic Energy
Chemicals and Chemists

Coal Mines
Environment
*Environmental pesticide control
Environmental Protection Agency
Environmental Quality Council
Hazard
Hazardous Agents
*Hazardous Materials Transportation
Narcotics
Noise Control
Nuclear Agents
Ocean Dumping
Occupational Safety and Health
Poisons
Radiation
Serums, Toxins, and Viruses
Solid Waste Disposal
*Toxic Mixtures or Substances
Water Pollution Prevention and Control

The *Code of Federal Regulations* (CFR) also has 50 titles which follow closely, but not exactly the *U.S. Code*. Following are some relevant titles:

7. Agriculture
15. Commerce and Foreign Trade
16. Commercial Practices
21. Food and Drugs
27. Alcohol, Tobacco Products, and Firearms
40. Protection of Environment
42. Public Health
45. Public Welfare
49. Transportation

There are numerous acts in addition to the ones listed in this section which may contain law pertinent to toxicology. Examples are:

Atomic Energy Act of 1954
Comprehensive Alcohol and Alcohol Prevention, Treatment, and Rehabilitation Act of 1970
Comprehensive Drug Abuse Prevention and Control Act of 1970
Dangerous Cargo Act
Egg Products Inspection Act
Fair Packaging and Labeling Act
Federal Caustic Poison
Federal Meat Inspection Act
Federal Mine Safety and Health Act
Federal Water Pollution Control Act
Flammable Fabrics Acts

Marine Mammal Protection Act of 1972
Marine Protection, Research and Sanctuaries Act of 1972
Ports and Waterways Safety Act
Public Health Service Act
Uranium Mill Tailings Radiation Control Act
Water Quality Improvement Act

Changes in important acts are often reflected in *Compilation of Selected Acts within the Jurisdiction of the Committee on Interstate and Foreign Commerce* (e), which is published every session of Congress. Legislative histories of various bills and acts provide valuable background materials and insight into rationale for law appearing in the form it finally does.

CIS/Annual: Index to Congressional Publications and Public Laws (f) published by Congressional Information Service, Inc. catalogs, abstracts, and indexes publications issues by Congress, as well as legislative histories.

Good discussions of legislation may be found in textbooks such as Cassaret & Doul and Sax, and in Congressional hearings and legislative histories.

Government Institutes, Inc., P.O. Box 5918, Washington DC 20014 is an active publisher in the environmental law field. They publish numerous books of interest to the toxicologist involved in regulations, sponsor conferences and offer courses.

One should never neglect to contact the organizations responsible for administration of the laws to get a more realistic picture of regulations. The newspapers, too, devote substantial space to environmental health regulations.

References

(a) *US statutes at large*. Washington, DC. Government Printing Office.

(b) *US code*. Washington, DC. Government Printing Office.

(c) *Federal Register*. Washington, DC. Office of the Federal Register.

(d) *Code of Federal Regulations*. Washington, DC. Office of the Federal Register.

(e) *Compilation of Selected Acts within the Jurisdiction of the Committee on Interstate and Foreign Commerce*. Washington, DC. Government Printing Office.

(f) *CIS/Annual. Part I: Abstracts of congressional publications and Legislative Histories. Part II: Index to Congressional Publications and Public Laws.* Washington, DC. Congressional Information Service.

695. *Clean Air Act* [PL 88-206, 1963]

Requires compilation of criteria documents for air pollutants. Sets national ambient air quality standards, standards for sources that create air pollution, for the emission of noxious air pollutants, and for motor vehicles, including aircraft. Primary responsibility for air pollution control is set with state and local governments with EPA responsible for the overall administration of the act. Amendments of 1970, 1977 allowed states additional time to meet standards.

696. *Clean Water Act of 1977* [PL 95-217, 1977]

Amends the Federal Water Pollution Control Act of 1972. Provides long-term funding for the municipal sewage treatment construction grant program. Limits pollution from industrial and municipal sources. Emphasizes the importance of controlling toxic pollutants that endanger public health. Encourages industry to experiment with the treatment of wastewater and sludge. Allows Federal and State governments to recover their costs in mitigating damages from spills of oil and other hazardous substances. Designed to make our water "fishable" and "swimmable."

697. *Consumer Product Safety Act* [PL 92-573, 1972]

To protect the public against unreasonable risks of injury associated with consumer products, to develop safety standards, and to promote research into causes and prevention of product related deaths, illness, and injuries.

698. *Controlled Substances Act* [PL 91-513, 1970]

"To amend the Public Health Service Act and other laws to provide increased research into, and prevention of, drug abuse and drug dependence, to provide for treatment and rehabilitation of drug abusers and drug dependent persons; and to strengthen existing law enforcement authority in the field of drug abuse."

699. *Federal Food, Drug, and Cosmetic Act* [52 Stat. 1040, 1938]

Replaced the 1960 Food and Drug Law. Required new drugs to be proven safe before marketing. Amended many times to cover regulation of food additives, color additives, therapeutic devices. The 1962 Drug Amendments for the first time required the manufacturer to prove safety *and* efficacy (Kefauver-Harris). The Delaney Clause of the 1958 Food Additives Amendment ruled that additives which are found to cause cancer in man or animals shall not be considered safe.

700. *Federal Hazardous Substances Act* [PL 86-613, 1960]

Included within the jurisdiction of this act are household products not covered by either the Federal Food, Drug, and Cosmetic Act or FIFRA.

701. *Federal Insecticide, Fungicide, and Rodenticide Act* [61 Stat. 163]

Regulates all pesticides marketed in the United States. Registration and toxicity studies of pesticides are required. Safety and efficiency studies must be provided. Labeling requirements are outlined.

702. *Hazardous Materials Transportation Act* [PL 93-633, 1975]

''To regulate commerce by improving the protections afforded the public against risks connected with the transportation of hazardous materials.''

703. *Lead-Based Paint Poison Prevention Act* [PL 91-695, 1971]

Intended to prevent poisoning of children by lead. Grants are authorized for detection and treatment of poisoning. Lead is regulated in various consumer items such as cooking utensils. Use of lead-based paint is restricted in residential structures.

704. *Noise Control Act of 1972* [PL 92-574, 1972]

Provides EPA with the mandate to find solutions to the problems of environmental noise which ''presents a growing danger to the health and welfare of the nation's population.'' EPA sets standards on noise levels for machinery and equipment.

705. *Occupational Safety and Health Act of 1970* [PL 91-596, 1970]

''To assure safe and healthful working conditions for working men and women; by authorizing enforcement of the standards developed under the Act; by assisting and encouraging the states in their efforts to assure safe and healthful working conditions; by providing for research, information, education, and training in the field of occupational safety and health.'' This act established NIOSH.

706. *National Environmental Policy Act of 1969 (NEPA)* [PL 91-190, 1970]

This act declares a national environmental policy and is the basis for establishment of environmental impact statements, which Federal agencies are required to prepare for all ''Federal actions significantly affecting the quality of the human environment.'' The statements should outline:

  i) the environmental impact on the proposed action.
  ii) any adverse environmental effects which cannot be avoided should the proposal be implemented.
  iii) alternatives to the proposed action.
  iv) the relationship between local short-term uses of man's environment and the maintenance and enhancement of long-term productivity.
  v) any irreversible and irretrievable commitments of resources which would be involved in the proposed action should it be implemented.''

NEPA is also responsible for the creation of the Council on Environmental Quality (CEQ), which, among other duties, reviews programs and develops and recommends policies to the President to promote improved environmental quality. CEQ also assists the President in the preparation of an annual Environmental Quality Report.

707. *Poison Prevention Packaging Act of 1970* [PL 91-601, 1970]

Administered by the Consumer Product Safety Commission (CPSC) who is authorized to set standards for the packaging of hazardous household products. Pesticides are not covered in this act. Intended to protect children from harm resulting from improperly packaged dangerous substances.

708. *Radiation Control for Health and Safety Act of 1968* [PL 90-602, 1968]

Amends the Public Health Service Act to provide for the protection of the public health from radiation emissions from electronic products. An important part of this act requires establishment of performance standards for certain radiation-producing electronic devices.

709. *Resource Conservation and Recovery Act of 1976* [PL 94-580]

Amends the 1965 Solid Waste Disposal Act and federally regulates solid waste. "To provide technical and financial assistance for the development of management plans and facilities for the recovery of energy and other resources from discarded materials, and to regulate the management of hazardous waste." Administered by EPA through their Office of Solid Waste. Fines are authorized for violation of any waste disposal regulations promulgated.

710. *Safe Drinking Water Act* [PL 93-523, 1974]

Sets standards for drinking water to protect the public health. Research is to be conducted relating to the causes, diagnosis, treatment, control, and prevention of diseases and impairments of man resulting directly or indirectly from contaminants in water. The states will file annual program plans outlining the exact manner in which they will conform to the national standards.

711. *Toxic Substances Control Act* [PL 94-469, 1976]

". . . empowers the federal government to control and even stop production or use of chemical substances that may present an unreasonable risk of injury to health or environment. Manufacturers must give notice of plans to produce a new chemical or to market a significant new use for an old chemical. Producers may also be required to test selected chemicals or to report production quantities, uses, physical, chemical, and biological properties, and other information necessary for hazard assessment. In addition, the law requires recordkeeping and disclosure of significant health effects of dangerous chemicals.'' [from the *Annual Report to the Council on Environmental Quality*, 1977]. This law is administered by the Environmental Protection Administration.

PART IV

INTERNATIONAL ACTIVITIES

Toxic substances are of worldwide concern and although this guide is concentrating on American sources and activities, the toxicologist should be acquainted with some of the major international activities, especially those in which the United States is involved.

The export of hazardous technology (in the form of agricultural chemicals, drugs, etc.) by industrialized nations to underdeveloped countries is an issue of concern, whether or not the importing country recognizes the hazards and whether or not it is willing to accept recognizable risks attending technological advances. National regulatory actions do not necessarily place any restrictions on imports/exports.

In addition to foreign commerce, the global community is affected by phenomena such as acid rain, stratospheric ozone depletion by chlorofluorocarbons, and the dumping of wastes in the ocean. Air-water-land pollution need not obey national boundaries.

Issues of data exchange, trade secrecy, and confidentiality, which have a long way to go toward resolution in this country, reach terrifying proportions when one considers the international scene. Free flow of information between countries is essential if we are to achieve standardization and uniformity (if these are indeed desirable) in nomenclature, good laboratory practice, and testing protocols.

The 1978 meeting in Stockholm, *International Meeting on the Control of Toxic Substances with Special Regard to Environmental Chemicals* identified the needs for toxic chemicals control within countries and encouraged international cooperation. The meeting was attended by 16 countries and 6 international organizations.

The following section lists international organizations, committees, etc. and 1 data network (*ECDIN*). A sampling of non-USA legislation, with dates of enactment, is also included. These laws are all akin to TSCA in the respect that they attempt to control hazardous/toxic chemicals. The approaches in terms of data reporting, terminology, responsibility for hazard assessment (government or industry), are variable, as are the means of implementation.

Chapter 17

Organizations—International

712. *Environmental Chemicals Data and Information Network (ECDIN)*
Joint Research Centre
Commission of the European Communities (CEC)
1-21020 Ispra (Varese), Italy

This system stores information on heavily manufactured and highly toxic chemicals. Over 100 data fields in some 11 categories (e.g., chemical nomenclature, chemical structure, physical and chemical properties, use and disposal, effects on the environment, etc.) have been identified. ECDIN is still in its pilot phase and information on public availability may be requested from the above address.

713. *European Economic Community (EEC)*
200 Rue de la Loi, B-1049 Brussels, Belgium

Aimed at promoting economic harmony among member states of the community. In June 1979 the EEC adopted the *Sixth Amendment* to the 1967 *Directive on Packaging and Labeling of Dangerous Substances*. This law corresponds somewhat to TSCA in that it requires notification by manufacturers of new chemicals in commerce. There are differences, however, in the method of notification as there are in approaches to testing. The 6th Amendment can only be implemented by having member countries pass legislation.

714. *Food and Agricultural Organization (FAO)*
Via delle Terme de Caracalla, 00100 Rome, Italy
North American Liason Office:
1776 F Street NW, Washington DC 20457

Part of the United Nations, the FAO seeks to raise world-wide nutrition levels and improve production and distribution of food and farm products. It is attempting to harmonize requirements for the registration of pesticides and formulate guidelines for environmental hazard assessment.

715. *Inter-Governmental Maritime Consultative Organization*
101-104 Picadilly, London W1V OAE, United Kingdom

An agency of the United Nations, which encourages intergovernmental cooperation in shipping, maritime safety, and prevention of ocean pollution. Has developed conventions for the prevention of pollution by ships carrying harmful chemicals, by sewage and garbage, and by the dumping of wastes.

716. *International Agency for Research on Cancer (IARC)*
150 Cours Albert Thomas, F 69008, Lyon, France

IARC is a part of WHO. IARC brings together experts on the carcinogenicity of various chemicals or classes of chemicals to help determine and evaluate the open scientific literature relating to the carcinogenic hazard of chemicals to man. IARC collaborates with NCI on various ventures.

717. *International Atomic Energy Agency*
Vienna International Centre
PO Box 100, Wagramerstrasse 5, A-1400 Vienna, Austria

Both promotes peaceful uses of atomic energy and establishes health and safety standards. Publishes *Nuclear Fusion* and *Atomic Energy Review*.

718. *International Commission on Radiological Protection*
Clifton Ave., Sutton Surrey SM2 5PU England

Considers principles of radiation protection and formulates advice or regulations for specific countries.

719. *International Labour Organization (ILO)*
4 Route des Morillons, CH-1211 Geneva 22, Switzerland
Washington Branch Address:
1750 New York Avenue NW, Washington, DC 20006

Promotes the well-being of workers throughout the world. Builds a code of labor standards. Among programs of particular importance to toxicology are the *International Occupational Safety and Health Information Centre (CIS)* or *Centre International d'Informations de securite et d'hygiene du travail, the International Occupational Safety and Health*

Hazard Alert System, and the *International Program for the Improvement of Working Conditions and Environment.*

720. *International Occupational Safety and Health Information Centre (CIS)*
International Labour Organization
CH-1211 Geneva 22, Switzerland
Washington Branch Address:
1750 New York Avenue NW, Washington, DC 20006

Collects, organizes and distributes information on worker protection from industrial hazards. Has developed a computerized data base system (*CISILO*) from which *CIS Abstracts* is published.

721. *International Register of Potentially Toxic Chemicals (IRPTC)*
IRPTC/UNEP
Palais des Nations
1210 Geneva, Switzerland
USA National Correspondent:
Dr. Marilyn Bracken
Director, Office of Program Integration and Information (TS-793)
Office of Pesticides and Toxic Substances
Environmental Protection Agency
Washington, DC 20460

IRPTC collects information on all potentially toxic chemicals and has established contacts with national and intergovernmental information systems and other organizations. IRPTC also operates a query-response service, which provides information on various aspects of toxicology. The *IRPTC Bulletin* contains current information on international activities. IRPTC is part of the *United Nations Environment Programme (UNEP)*. Recent IRPTC activities include completion of an "attributes study," which involved development of a list of attributes of chemicals that would help in evaluating their hazards and preparation of a list of priority chemicals.

722. *Organization for Economic Cooperation and Development (OECD)*
2 Rue Andre Pascal, 75775 Paris Cedex 16, France
Publications and Information Center:
OECD, Suite 1207, 1750 Pennsylvania Avenue NW, Washington, DC 20006

Promotes economic welfare in member countries. Important activities include the "Chemicals Testing Program," which is developing test guidelines, and the "Program on the Control of Chemicals," which is involved in 3 priority projects—good laboratory practices, data confidentiality, and an international glossary of terms. OECD's Council relating to the environment has passed numerous decisions, resolutions and recommendations on topics such as PCBs, mercury emissions, noise prevention, and transfrontier pollution. In 1974 OECD adopted the implementation of the "polluter-pays principle."

723. *United Nations Environment Programme (UNEP)*
P.O. Box 30552, Nairobi, Kenya

Coordinates and promotes international environmental cooperation. Three major program activities are 1. the *Global Monitoring System (GEMS)* 2. the *International Registry of Potentially Toxic Chemicals (IRPTC)* and 3. *INFOTERRA,* a decentralized international environmental information network employing referral of requests.

724. *World Health Organization (WHO)*
1211 Geneva 27, Switzerland
United States address:
525 23rd St, NW, Washington, DC 20036

The WHO Constitution states, "The objective of WHO shall be the attainment by all peoples of the highest possible level of health." Among its programs are the *Program on the Evaluation of the Effects of Chemicals on Health,* the *International Programme on Chemical Safety,* and the *Environmental Health Criteria Programme.*

Chapter 18

Representative Legislation—International

725. Canada: *Environmental Contaminants Act*—1975
726. France: *French Chemicals Control Act of 1977*—1977
727. Japan: *Chemical Substances Control Law of 1973*—1973
728. Norway: *Act Concerning the Control of Products Hazardous to Health and the Environment*—1976
729. Sweden: *Act on Products Hazardous to Health and the Environment*—1973
730. Switzerland: *Swiss Law on Trade in Toxic Substances*—1969
731. United Kingdom: *Health and Safety Act of 1974*—1974
732. EEC: *Sixth Amendment to the 1967 Directive on Packaging and Labeling of Dangerous Substances*—1979

PART V

EDUCATION

Toxicology education is still in its infancy. Compared to other scientific disciplines, there is a shortage of schools offering programs in toxicology and a consequent shortage of trained toxicologists. The following list of graduate programs in toxicology has been compiled by the Education Committee of the Society of Toxicology. There are no schools of toxicology as there are schools of law, medicine, etc. Instead there are programs, departments, interdepartmental curricula, divisions, etc. within schools of pharmacy, medicine, veterinary medicine, agriculture, public health, etc. Toxicology course offerings are on the increase in other scientific programs as well.

Aside from the university programs, there are short courses sponsored by numerous organizations including some of those listed in this book. The American Chemical Society, for instance, offers a three day course entitled "Toxicology for Chemists" as well as other pertinent courses. Government Institutes Inc., 4733 Bethesda Ave NW, Washington DC 20014 offers courses and seminars concentrating on regulatory matters, as does the Center for Energy and Environmental Management, P.O. Box 536, Fairfax, VA. EPA recently sponsored a course in Chemical Information Resources developed by Koba Associates Inc., Environmental Sciences Division, 2000 Florida Avenue NW, Washington DC 20009.

Chapter 19

Universities Offering
Graduate Programs in Toxicology

Compiled by the Education Committee of the Society of Toxicology

Note : * Indicates person who should be contacted for further information

F Indicates programs in forensic toxicology available

ALABAMA

733. Auburn University
Pharmacology & Toxicology
Dept. (F)
School of Pharmacy
Auburn, Alabama 36830
Dr. B. B. Williams*

734. Tuskegee Institute
Physiology & Pharmacology
Dept.
School of Veterinary Medicine
Tuskegee, Alabama 36088
Dr. R. R. Dalvi*

735. University of Alabama in Birmingham
Pharmacology Dept.
School of Medicine and School of Dentistry
University Station
Birmingham, Alabama 35294
Dr. Roy L. Mundy*

ARIZONA

736. University of Arizona
Toxicology Program
Tucson, Arizona 85271
Dr. J. Wesley Clayton*

737. University of Arizona
Dept. of Entomology
College of Agriculture
Tucson, Arizona 85721
Dr. George Ware*

ARKANSAS

738. University of Arkansas
College of Pharmacy
4301 West Markham
Little Rock, Arkansas 72201
Dr. C. Allen Bradley*

739. University of Arkansas for Medical Sciences
Interdisciplinary Toxicology
Graduate Program
4301 West Markham
Little Rock, Arkansas 72201
Dr. Donald E. McMillan*

CALIFORNIA

740. Loma Linda University
Dept. of Pharmacology
Loma Linda, California 92354
Dr. Allen Strother*

741. University of California at Davis
Environmental Toxicology Dept.
College of Agriculture and
Environmental Sciences
Davis, California 95616
Dr. James N. Seiber*

742. University of California at Davis
Graduate Group in
Pharmacology and Toxicology
Davis, California 95616
Dr. Theodore C. West*

743. University of California at San Francisco
Pharmacology & Experimental
Therapeutics Dept.
San Francisco, California 94143
Dr. C. H. Hine*

COLORADO

744. Colorado State University
Institute of Rural Environmental
Health
College of Veterinary Medicine
and Biomedical Sciences
Fort Collins, Colorado 80523
Dr. Walter W. Melvin, Jr.*

CONNECTICUT

745. University of Connecticut in Storrs
Pharmacology and Toxicology
Dept.
College of Pharmacy
U-92 Storrs, Connecticut 06268
Dr. Steven D. Cohen*

DISTRICT OF COLUMBIA

746. Georgetown University
Dept. of Pharmacology
3900 Reservoir Rd. N.W.
Washington, D.C. 20007
Dr. Frank G. Standaert*

747. Howard University (F)
Department of Pharmacology
College of Medicine
Washington, D.C. 20059
Dr. William L. West*

FLORIDA

748. Florida A and M University
Division of Pharmacology and
Toxicology
School of Pharmacy
Tallahassee, Florida 32307
Dr. William R. Primas*

GEORGIA

749. Medical College of Georgia
Pharmacology Dept.
College of Medicine/School of
Graduate Studies
Augusta, Georgia 30902
Dr. J. M. Kling*

IDAHO

750. Idaho State University
Pharmacology Dept.

College of Pharmacy-CD 210
Pocatello, Idaho 83209
Dr. Gary E. Isom*

ILLINOIS

751. Loyola University of Chicago
Pharmacology Dept.
Stritch School of Medicine
2160 South First Avenue
Maywood, Illinois 60153
Dr. Joseph R. Davis*

752. Northwestern University
Dept. of Pharmacology
Chicago, Illinois 60611
Dr. Toshio Narahashi*

753. University of Illinois/Medical Center
Medicinal Chemistry Dept.
College of Pharmacy
833 South Wood Street
P.O. Box 6998
Chicago, Illinois 60680
Dr. Michael Mimnaugh*

754. University of Illinois/Medical Center
Occupational & Environmental Health Dept.
School of Public Health
Chicago, Illinois 60680
Dr. Badi Boulos*

755. University of Illinois at Urbana-Champaign
College of Veterinary Medicine
Urbana, Illinois 61801
Dr. W. B. Buck*

INDIANA

756. Indiana University
Pharmacology and Toxicology Dept. (F)

School of Medicine
1100 West Michigan Street
Indianapolis, Indiana 46202
Dr. Robert B. Forney*

757. Purdue University
Interdepartmental Program in Toxicology
School of Health Sciences
West Lafayette, Indiana 47907
Dr. J. E. Christian*

758. Purdue University
Pharmacology and Toxicology Dept.
School of Pharmacy and Pharmacol. Sciences
West Lafayette, Indiana 47907
Dr. Roger P. Maickel*

IOWA

759. Iowa State University
Veterinary Pathology Dept.
College of Veterinary Medicine
Ames, Iowa 50011
Dr. W. Eugene Lloyd*

760. University of Iowa School of Medicine
Pharmacology Dept.
Iowa City, Iowa 52242
Dr. Thomas Tephly*

KANSAS

761. Kansas State University
Comparative Toxicology Laboratory
Manhattan, Kansas 66506
Dr. F. W. Oehme*

762. The University of Kansas Medical Center
Pharmacology Dept.
Kansas City, Kansas 66103
Dr. Curtis D. Klaassen*

169

763. **University of Kansas**
Pharmacology and Toxicology,
    Medicinal Chemistry Depts.
College of Pharmacy
Lawrence, Kansas 66044
    Dr. Duane G. Wenzel*

KENTUCKY

764. **University of Kentucky**
Graduate Center for Toxicology
Lexington, Kentucky 40546
    Dr. Wyman Dorough*

LOUISIANA

765. **L.S.U. Medical Center**
Dept. of Pharmacology
P.O. Box 33932
Shreveport, Louisiana 71130
    Dr. Joseph Marino*

766. **Northeast Louisiana
University**
Pharmacology and Toxicology
    Division
School of Pharmacy
Monroe, Louisiana 71209
    Dr. T. H. Eickholt*

767. **Tulane University**
Department of Pharmacology
School of Medicine
1430 Tulane Avenue
New Orleans, LA 70112
    Dr. William J. George*

768. **Tulane University**
Dept. of Environmental Health
    Science
School of Public Health
1430 Tulane Avenue
New Orleans, LA 70112
    Dr. LuAnn White*

MARYLAND

769. **Johns Hopkins University**
Dept. of Environmental Health
    Sciences
School of Hygiene & Public
    Health
Baltimore, Maryland 21205
    Dr. Robert J. Rubin*

770. **Johns Hopkins University**
School of Hygiene and Public
    Health
Baltimore, Maryland 21205
    Dr. Zoltan Annau*

771. **University of Maryland**
Pharmacology and Toxicology
    Dept.
School of Pharmacy
636 W. Lombard Street
Baltimore, Maryland 21201
    Dr. Gary M. Oderda*

772. **University of Maryland,
School of Medicine**
Dept. of Pathology (F)
Div. of Forensic Pathology
111 Penn Street
Baltimore, Maryland 21201
    Dr. Yale H. Caplan*

MASSACHUSETTS

773. **Harvard University**
Physiology Dept.
School of Public Health
665 Huntington Avenue
Boston, Massachusetts 02115
    Dr. A. H. Tashjian, Jr.*

774. **Massachusetts Institute of
Technology**
Nutrition and Food Science
Department

School of Sciences
Cambridge, Massachusetts
02139
Dr. Gerald Wogan*

775. Northeastern University
Program in Toxicology (F)
College of Pharmacy and Allied
Health Professions
360 Huntington Avenue
Boston, Massachusetts 02115
Dr. David Brown*

MICHIGAN

776. Michigan State University
Center of Environmental
Toxicology
East Lansing, Michigan 48824
Dr. J. B. Hook*

777. University of Michigan
Interdepartmental Program in
Toxicology
7533 School of Public Health
Ann Arbor, Michigan 48109
Dr. Rolf Hartung*

778. University of Michigan
Environmental and Industrial
Health Dept.
M7525 School of Public Health
Ann Arbor, Michigan 48109
Dr. Herbert H. Cornish*

779. Wayne State University
Department of Pharmacology
1400 Chrysler Drive
Detroit, Michigan 48202
Dr. R. T. Louis-Ferdinand*

MINNESOTA

780. University of Minnesota
Pharmacology Dept.

105 Millard Hall
Minneapolis, Minnesota 55455
Dr. M. W. Anders*

MISSISSIPPI

**781. University of Mississippi
Medical Center**
Pharmacology and Toxicology
Dept. (F)
2500 North State Street
Jackson, Mississippi 39216
Dr. William O. Berndt*

**782. University of Mississippi,
Oxford Campus**
Pharmacology Dept.
School of Pharmacy
University, Mississippi 38677
Dr. Lawrence W. Masten*

MISSOURI

783. University of Missouri
Veterinary Anatomy-Physiology
College of Veterinary Medicine
Columbia, Missouri 65201
Dr. Gary D. Osweiler*

NEBRASKA

**784. University of Nebraska
Medical Center**
Dept. of Pharmacodynamics and
Toxicology
Omaha, Nebraska 68105
Dr. Craig Schnell*

NEW HAMPSHIRE

785. Dartmouth Medical School
Pharmacology & Toxicology
Dept.
Hanover, New Hampshire 03755
Dr. Roger P. Smith*

NEW JERSEY

786. **College of Medicine and Dentistry of New Jersey**
Pharmacology Dept.
Graduate School of Biomedical Sciences
100 Bergen Street
Newark, New Jersey 07103
Dr. Sheldon B. Gertner*

NEW YORK

787. **Albany Medical College**
Center of Experimental Pathology & Toxicology
Albany, New York 12208
Dr. Rejender Abraham*

788. **Cornell University**
Field of Toxicology
Ithaca, New York 14853
Dr. Christopher F. Wilkinson*

789. **New York University**
Dept. of Environmental Medicine
New York, New York 10003
Dr. Morton Lippman*

790. **New York University Medical Center**
Dept. of Environmental Medicine
New York, New York 10016
Dr. Roy E. Albert*

791. **New York State College of Veterinary Medicine**
Dept. of Physiology, Biochemistry, and Pharmacology
Ithaca, New York 14853
Dr. Arthur Aronson*

792. **Roswell Park Memorial Institute**
New York State Department of Health
Buffalo, New York 14263
Dr. Harold Box*

793. **Saint Johns University**
Pharmaceutical Sciences Dept.
College of Pharmacy and Allied Health Professions
Grand Central and Utopia Parkways
Jamaica, New York 11439
Dr. Vincent dePaul Lynch*

794. **State University of New York at Buffalo**
School of Pharmacy
H347, Hochstetter Complex
Buffalo, New York 14260
Dr. Nathan Back*

795. **University of Rochester**
School of Medicine and Dentistry
Rochester, New York 14642
Dr. Victor G. Laties*

NORTH CAROLINA

796. **Duke University School of Medicine**
Pulmonary Medicine Division
Medicine Department
Durham, North Carolina 27710
Dr. William Lynn*

797. **North Carolina State University**
Entomology, Toxicology Depts.
College of Agriculture
Raleigh, North Carolina 27607
Dr. Frank E. Guthrie*

798. University of North Carolina
Curriculum in Toxicology
Dept. Biochemistry and
Nutrition
Medical School
Chapel Hill, NC 27514
Dr. David Holbrook*

799. University of North Carolina
Environmental Pathology
Department of Pathology
Medical School
Chapel Hill, NC 27514
Dr. Joe W. Gresham*

NORTH DAKOTA

800. North Dakota State University
Pharmacology and Toxicology
Dept. (F)
College of Pharmacy
Fargo, North Dakota 58102
Dr. N. G. S. Rao*

OHIO

**801. Children's Hospital Medical
Center**
Dept. of Pediatrics
Cincinnati, Ohio 45229
Dr. Ernest F. Zimmerman*

802. Cleveland State University
Chemistry Department
Euclid Avenue
Cleveland, Ohio 44115
Dr. Julius Kerkay*

803. Ohio State University
Pharmacology Division
College of Pharmacy
500 W. 12th Avenue
Columbus, Ohio 43210
Dr. Ralf G. Rahwan*

804. Ohio State University
Veterinary Physiology,
Pharmacology Depts.
Veterinary Medicine
1900 Coffey Road
Columbus, Ohio 43210
Dr. Roger A. Yeary*

805. University of Cincinnati
Environmental Health Dept. (F)
College of Medicine—Kettering
Laboratory
3223 Eden Avenue
Cincinnati, Ohio 45267
Dr. Paul Hammond*

**806. University of Cincinnati
Medical Center**
College of Pharmacy (Mail Loc.
4)
Cincinnati, Ohio 45267
Dr. Verna L. Armstrong*

OKLAHOMA

**807. University of Oklahoma
College of Pharmacy**
Pharmacodynamic & Toxicology
Dept.
644 NE 14th Street HSC
Oklahoma City, Oklahoma
73190
Dr. Joseph A. Rieger*

OREGON

808. Oregon State University
Pharmacology and Toxicology
Dept.
School of Pharmacy
Corvallis, Oregon 97331
Dr. Robert E. Larson*

809. Oregon State University
Environmental Health Sciences
Center

Corvallis, Oregon 97331
Dr. Ian J. Tinsley*

PENNSYLVANIA

810. Duquesne University
School of Pharmacy (F)
Pittsburgh, Pennsylvania 15219
Dr. Charles L. Winek*

811. Philadelphia College of
Pharmacy and Science
Biological Sciences Dept.
43rd Street, Kingsessing Mall
Philadelphia, Pennsylvania
19104
Dr. Gary Lage*

812. Temple University School of
Pharmacy
Medicinal Chemistry and
Pharmaceutical Dept. (F)
3307 N. Broad Street
Philadelphia, Pennsylvania
19140
Dr. Tully J. Speaker*

813. Thomas Jefferson University
Pharmacology Dept.
1020 Locust Street
Philadelphia, Pennsylvania
19107
Dr. Anthony J. Triolo*

814. University of Pennsylvania
Dept. of Pharmacology and
Toxicology (F)
3800 Spruce Street
Philadelphia, Pennsylvania
19104
Dr. Carl E. Aronson*

815. University of Pittsburgh
School of Public Health
Indl. Environmental Hlth. Sci

Pittsburgh, Pennsylvania 15261
Dr. Y. Allarie*

RHODE ISLAND

816. University of Rhode Island
Pharmacology and Toxicology
Dept.
College of Pharmacy
Kingston, Rhode Island 02881
Dr. Paul Carroll*

TENNESSEE

817. The University of Tennessee
Center for the Health Sciences
College of Pharmacy
Drug & Material Toxicology
Dept.
874 Union Avenue
Memphis, Tennessee 38163
Dr. W. H. Lawrence*

818. The University of Tennessee
Center for the Health Sciences
(F)
College of Medicine
Pathology Dept.
3 North Dunlap Street
Memphis, Tennessee 38163
Dr. David T. Stafford*

819. The University of Tennessee
College of Liberal Arts
Environmental Toxicology
Graduate Program in Ecology
Knoxville, Tennessee 37916
Dr. Lena B. Brattsten*

820. Vanderbilt University
Center in Toxicology
Department of Biochemistry
Nashville, Tennessee 37232
Dr. F. P. Guengerich*

TEXAS

821. Texas A & M University
Veterinary Physiology,
Pharmacology Depts.
College of Veterinary Medicine
College Station, Texas 77843
Dr. J. D. McCrady*

822. The University of Texas
College of Pharmacy
Department of Pharmacology
Austin, Texas 78712
Dr. Alan B. Combs*

823. University of Texas
Dept. of Pharmacology
Dallas, Texas 75235
Dr. George B. Weiss*

824. University of Texas Health Science Center
Division of Toxicology
Medical School
P.O. Box 20708
Houston, Texas 77025
Dr. Sheldon D. Murphy*

825. The University of Texas Health Science Center
Pharmacology Department
7703 Floyd Curl Drive
San Antonio, Texas 78284
Dr. William B. Stavinoha*

826. The University of Texas Medical Branch
Graduate School of Biomedical Sciences (F)
Galveston, Texas 77550
Toxicology Program
Dr. J. Palmer Saunders*
Pathology Dept.
Dr. Edward S. Reynolds, Jr.*
Pharmacology and Toxicology
Dr. Walter J. Decker*

Preventive Medicine and
Community Health Dept.
Dr. Marvin S. Legator*

UTAH

827. University of Utah
Colleges of Pharmacy and Medicine
Salt Lake City, Utah 84132
Graduate Studies in Toxicology
Dr. James W. Gibb*
Center for Human Toxicology
Dr. Bryan S. Finkle*

828. Utah State University
Interdepartmental Curriculum
College of Agriculture
UMC 56
Logan, Utah 84322
Dr. R. P. Sharma*

VIRGINIA

829. Virginia Commonwealth University
Pharmacology Dept. (F)
Medical College of Virginia
Richmond, Virginia 23298
Dr. Joseph F. Borzelleca*

WASHINGTON

830. University of Washington School of Medicine
Dept. of Pharmacology (F)
Seattle, Washington 98105
Dr. Ted Loomis*

831. Washington State University
Pharmacology Dept.
College of Pharmacy
Pullman, Washington 99163
Dr. W. E. Johnson*

WEST VIRGINIA

832. West Virginia University
W.V.U. School of Medicine
Medical Center
Pharmacology and Toxicology
Dept.
Morgantown, West Virginia
26506
Dr. William W. Fleming*

WISCONSIN

833. The Medical College of Wisconsin
Pharmacology and Toxicology
Dept.

P.O. Box 26509
Milwaukee, Wisconsin 53226
Dr. James M. Fujimoto*

834. University of Wisconsin
School of Pharmacy
425 N. Charter Street
Madison, Wisconsin 53706
Dr. Richard E. Peterson*

835. University of Wisconsin
Center for Environmental
Toxicology
1550 Linden Drive
Madison, Wisconsin 53706
Dr. Ronald D. Hinsdill*

We recognize that this list is probably incomplete and we welcome additions and corrections. Inclusion on the list does not constitute endorsement by SOT any more than exclusion constitutes a lack of endorsement.

PART VI

INFORMATION HANDLING

Chapter 20

Information Handling

Articles and books on toxicology information resources (including data bases) are located in this category. These items concern themselves with the handling of toxicology information rather than toxicology as a scientific entity. This list should be especially useful to the librarian, information specialist, or other professional involved in information collection, organization, dissemination, or retrieval.

This entire bibliography is, in a sense, concerned with information handling and the toxicologist would do well to familiarize himself with literature that stresses ways of systematically approaching the mass of information in toxicology. Creation and use of data bases is bound to increase and optimal use of systems requires that the user be properly trained and keep up with changes as reflected in the literature.

In addition to the titles in the serials section of this bibliography which have emphasized scientific aspects but may contain information handling aspects of the subject, the following periodicals are worth consulting on a regular basis:

Database. Weston, CT. Online. 1978—

Drug Information Journal. East Hanover, NJ. Information Association. 6, 1972—[Continues *Drug Information Bulletin*]

Journal of Chemical Information and Computer Sciences. Washington, DC. American Chemical Society. 15, 1975—[Continues *Journal of Chemical Documentation*]

Online. Weston CT. Online. 1, 1976—

Online Review. Medford, NJ. Learned Information.

Special Libraries. New York. Special Libraries Association. 1, 1910—

The following indexing and abstracting tools, when searched under the appropriate subject headings will lead to literature appearing in journals such as those aforementioned:

Information Science Abstracts. Philadelphia. Documentation Abstracts. 1966—

Library Literature. Bronx, NY. HW Wilson. 1936—

Library and Information Science Abstracts. London. Library Association. 1969—

NTIS Weekly Government Abstracts on Library and Information Sciences. National Technical Information Service.

The Cosmides symposium specifically addresses the entire question of information handling. In coming years, professional groups should include information sessions in their programs so that their members can become aware of at least the capabilities of existing and projected computer systems. Current research builds on past research and in order to take fullest advantage of work that has been done earlier and to avoid duplication of effort, all scientific investigations should be preceded by a comprehensive literature search. The materials in this section should aid in the actual searching or help the requester (assuming he is different from the searcher) understand what tools are available for searching and how they may best be utilized.

836. Bac R. A comparative study by the PDR of toxicology information retrieval from online literature databases. *Online* 4(2):29–33, Apr 1980.

> The Toxicology Data Committee of the Pharma Documentation Ring (PDR) examined literature retrieved from four data bases in response to four questions. 58% of all the references retrieved appeared in only 1 data base. Overlap is analyzed and recommendations are given for similar comparative studies and for the coding of toxicological information.

837. Bawden D. Chemical toxicology searching. *Database* 2(2):11–18. Jun 1979.

> Detailed article on use of on-line bibliographic data bases. Discusses Chemical Abstracts, BIOSIS, TOXLINE, MEDLINE, Excerpta Medica, Science Citation Index. RINGDOC and NTIS are also mentioned in less detail. Typical information on data bases includes coverage, indexing, user aids, chemical substance searching, toxic effect searching and searching hints. Summary tables indicate search features. Particularly useful is a section on "combinations of data bases," which suggests appropriate data bases to use for different areas of toxicology.

838. Bernstein HJ, Andrews LC. The NIH-EPA chemical information system. *Database* 2(1):35–49, March 1979.

The NIH-EPA system is comprised of a variety of data bases most useful for chemical identification and characterization. One subsystem, the Oil & Hazardous Materials Technical Assistance Data System, may be particularly useful in obtaining data on toxicity and hazards on some 1000 substances that are transported in large quantities. NIH-EPA offers RTECS which is also available from NLM. The article provides sample printouts.

839. Bracken MC. Information systems for predicting chemical hazards. *J Environ Pathol Toxicol* 2:133–40, 1978.

A glimpse into the future. The Chemical Substances Information Network (CSIN) is described. This network will build upon existing systems and support research and decision making activities.

840. *Chemical Information Resource Handbook.* Washington, DC. Koba Associates. 1980.

Produced under EPA contract for the Office of Pesticides and Toxic Substances, this handbook describes the more important chemical information resources accessible through government and privately. The majority of the resources are data bases. For most of these, information is provided on the data base's scope, means of access and cost. Sample searches and output are also provided. Both existing and proposed systems have been included.

841. Comstock EG. Drug information resources for treatment of acute drug overdose. *Drug Inform J* 9(2/3):81–88, May/Sep 1975.

A somewhat general but interesting article on the problems of obtaining comprehensive and timely information for treatment of drug overdose. Good discussion on variation in scope of information in PDR. Author provides a list of nine items which should ideally be available on all package inserts in order to "develop a rational approach to treatment."

842. Cosmides GJ, Ed. *Symposium on the Handling of Toxicological Information.* Bethesda, MD. Department of Health, Education and Welfare. 1978. [Available from NTIS—PB-283 164]

"This 1976 symposium was organized to consider developments over the last decade in the handling of toxicological information, the present state of information handling and future requirements. The proceedings, consisting of 33 papers and ensuing discussion, are organized within the symposium's structure of panels covering sources of toxicological information, interorganizational requirements for legislation, decision-making, and special user groups (such as industry, the news media, and consumers), and recommendations."

843. Fisher KD, Carr CJ. Consumer views on information resources in toxicology. *Drug Inform J* 9(2/3):64–72, May/Sep 1975.

Concentrates on the difficulties in accessing toxicology information. Stresses the interdisciplinary nature of the field and using the specific example of iodine the article traces the variety of sources which may need to be consulted.

844. Gerstner HB, Huff JE. Unique sources of drug toxicology information. *Drug Inform J* 9(2/3):161–167, May/Sep 1975.

Describes the services of the Information Division of the Oak Ridge National Laboratory (ORNL), especially the Toxicology Information Response Center (TIRC).

845. Gillespie CJ. Drug information services. *Adv Pharmacol Chemother* 15:51–85, 1978.

Although this article's intent is to deal specifically with drug information, the services covered are very relevant to toxicology. There is an emphasis on capabilities, advantages and disadvantages of numerous computer systems.

846. Heller SR, Milne, GWA. NIH-EPA Chemical information system. *Database* 2(3):68–79, Sep 1979.

A detailed discussion of this unique system of nonbibligraphic data bases. Sample printouts are included.

847. Huleatt RS. Product safety literature searches. *Database* 1(2):26–33, Dec 1978.

The Armour Research Center has developed a standard strategy for searching the NLM data bases for the safety of chemical substances.

848. Huleatt RS. Online use of chemical abstracts. *Database* 2(4):11–21, Dec 1979.

A description of the various Chemical Abstracts databases, their capabilities, discussion of vendors. Material on future possibilities for CODEN, CAS Registry numbers, back-issue coverage.

849. Johnson SW, Rader RA. Information retrieval for the safety evaluation of cosmetic products. *Special Libraries* 69(5/6):206–214, May/Jun 1978.

The authors, with the Gillette Medical Evaluation Laboratories Information Center describe their procedures and tools used for determining the safety of their products. Tables of sources include 1. source of nomenclature, 2. repeatedly used references, 3. most frequently used sources of current events information, and 4. ongoing safety reviews. Section on government agencies. A useful reference for anyone involved in accessing cosmetics information.

850. Kasperko J. Online chemical dictionaries: A comparison. *Database* 2(3):24–35, Sep 1979.

Compares CHEMNAME, CHEMDEX, and CHEMLINE files, strengths, weaknesses, and special features.

851. Kissman H. Information retrieval in toxicology. *Ann Rev Pharmacol Toxicol* 20:285–305, 1980.

Although this article is directed to toxicologists and pharmacologists, it is also of great practical value to librarians and information specialists. Problems of and sources in toxicology information are fully discussed. Storage and delivery systems are stressed. Over 100 references plus a table of the highest cited journals in TOXLINE.

852. Kremin M. Chemical search reference tools. *Database* 2(1):50–52, Mar 1979.

An annotated list of 10 basic reference tools dealing with chemistry, chemical nomenclature, and toxicology.

853. Marquart RG, Marquart LM, Mintz SA, Heller SR, Milne GWA. The NIH/EPA CIS Federal Register Notices search system. *Online* 4(2):45–49, Apr 1980.

The authors describe a valuable tool for the computer searching of federal regulations by chemical or chemical fragment. Some available search parameters are EPA/Pesticides codes, EPA pollution regulation, FDA codes, FDA drug dosage codes, etc.

854. McGill JR, Heller SR, Milne GWA. A computer-based toxicology search system. *J Environ Pathol Toxicol* 2(2):539–551, 1978.

A fairly detailed discussion of the NIOSH-RTECS interactive computer search system.

855. Oxman MA, Kissman HM. The toxicology data bank. *J Chem Inform Comp Sci* 16(1):19–21, 1976.

A description of TDB.

856. Sewell W. *Guide to Drug Information.* Hamilton, Ill., Drug Intelligence Publications, 1976.

A comprehensive look at drug information. Sources of information from toxic effects, adverse reactions, and drug interactions are scattered

throughout this book. In considering the overall problem of drug information, this text should supplement this syllabus. Useful tables include
one which compares drug handbooks and indicates what types of information may be extracted from each.

857. Statistics on the environment and on occupational safety and health In *A
Framework for Planning U.S. Federal Statistics for the 1980's.*
Washington. Office of Federal Statistical Policy and Standards. 1978.
[Available from GPO–003-005-00183-2)

Looks at the Federal Government's efforts at data collection and statistical analysis in areas of air, water, occupational safety and health,
energy, pesticides, toxics, and populations at risk. Discusses statistical
information as it exists, plus issues, problems, and areas that need
strengthening.

858. Temple AR. Poison control centers: Prospects and capabilities. *Ann Rev
Pharmacol Toxicol* 17:215–222, 1977.

A description of the poison control center program in this country, its
limitations and future needs. There is a section on toxicology information resources.

859. Tchobanoff JB. The data bases of food. *Online* 4(1):20–25, Jan 1980.

A survey of files for searching all aspects of foods, including their
toxicology.

PART VII

JOURNAL ARTICLES

Chapter 21

Journal Articles

Journal articles are usually the primary source for scientific information. Most of the other publications in this guide, such as books, rely on journals articles for their ultimate content. The journal article is, perhaps, the first step in the formal transfer of scientific information. The material is timely, ever-changing and ever-growing. This part of the guide is meant to supplement the reference resources in a few topics of interest. The articles selected have generally been recent (published since 1977) review articles in English. The categories, which do not precisely correspond to the categories of books, are as follows:

A. Biotoxins
B. Carcinogenesis, Mutagenesis, Teratogenesis
C. Cosmetics
D. Drugs
E. Environmental Toxicology
F. Food
G. Legislation, Regulations, and Societal Issues
H. Metals
I. Occupational Health and Industrial Hygiene
J. Pesticides
K. Radiation

Consulting abstracts, indexes, current awareness tools, and data bases will lead the reader to the most current journal articles.

There are duplicates of journal citations appearing among the categories to facilitate scanning.

Biotoxins

860. Arbuthnott JP. Role of exotoxins in bacterial pathogenicity. *J Appl Bacteriol* 44(3):329–345, Jun 1978.

861. Bababunmi EA, Thabrew I, Bassir O. Aflatoxin-induced coagulopathy in different nutritionally classified animal species. *Worl Rev Nutr Diet* 34:161–181, 1980.

862. Barnard EA, Dolly JO, Lang B, Lo M, Shorr RG. Application of specifically acting toxins to the detection of functional components common to peripheral and central synapses. *Adv Cytopharmacol* 3:409–434, 1979.

863. Beckstead JW, Rawson RD, Giles WS. Review of bite mark evidence. *J Am Dent Assoc* 99(1):69–74, Jul 1979.

864. Berry LJ. The mediation of endotoxemic effects. *Toxicon* (Suppl 1):869–887, 1978.

865. Bikhazi GB. Endotoxemia. *Middle East J Anaesthesiol* 5(5):357–368, Oct 1979.

866. Brown DA. Neurotoxins and the ganglionic (C6) type of nicotinic receptor. *Adv Cytopharmacol* 3:225–230, 1979.

867. Campadelli-Fiume G. Amanitins in virus research. *Arch Virol* 58(1):1–13, 1978.

868. Chu FS. Mycotoxin-macromolecule bindings. *Toxicon* (Suppl 1):713–728, 1978,

869. Ciegler A. Fungi that produce mycotoxins: conditions and occurrence. *Mycopathologia* 65(1–3):5–11, Dec 18 1978.

870. Clement JF, Pietrusko RG. Pit viper snakebite envenomation in the United States. *Clin Toxicol* 14(5):515–538, 1979.

871. Costantino D. Mushroom poisoning in Italy. *Int J Artif Organs* 1(6):257–259, Nov 1978.

872. Dowdall MJ, Fohlman JP, Watts A. Presynaptic action of snake venom neurotoxins on cholinergic systems. *Adv Cytopharmacol* 3:63–76, 1979.

873. Erspamer V, Melchiorri P, Erspamer CF, Negri L. Polypeptides of the amphibian skin active on the gut and their mammalian counterparts. *Adv Exp Med Biol* 106:51–64, 1978.

874. Faulstich H. New aspects of amanita poisoning. *Klin Wochensch* 57(21):1143–1152, Nov 1979.

875. Foil LD, Norment BR. Envenomation by Loxosceles reclusa. *J Med Entomol* 16(1):18–25, Sep 1979.

876. Godman GC, Miranda AF. Cellular contractility and the visible effects of cytochalasin. *Front Biol* 46:277–429, 1978.

877. Gorio A, Mauro A. Mode of action of black widow spider venom on vertebrate neuromuscular junction. *Adv. Cytopharmacol* 3:129–140, 1979.

878. Gothe R, Kunze K, Hoogstraal H. The mechanisms of pathogenicity in the tick paralyses. *J Med Entomol* 16(5):357–369, Nov 23 1979.

879. Gurtoo HL, Dahms R, Vaught JB. Metabolism of a prototype mycotoxin, aflatoxin B1, and its genetic regulation. *Mycopathologia* 65(1–3):13–28, Dec 18 1978.

880. Habermann E, Fischer K. Apamin, a centrally acting neurotoxic peptide: binding and actions. *Adv Cytopharmacol* 3:387–394, 1979.

881. Harrison TE. Ergotaminism. *JACEP* 7(4):162–169, Apr 1978.

882. Hartmann GR, Richter H, Weiner EM, Zimmermann W. On the mechanism of action of the cytostatic drug anguidine and of the immunosuppressive agent ovalicin, two sesquiterpenes from fungi. *Planta Med* 34(3):231–252, Nov 1978.

883. Hayes AW. Biological activities of mycotoxins. *Mycopathologia* 65(1–3):29–41, Dec 18 1978.

884. Henney CS. The use of cytochalasins to probe the immunobiology of lymphocytes. *Front Biol* 46:191–215, 1978.

885. Hiserodt JC, Granger GA. The human lymphotoxin system. *J Reticuloendothel Soc* 24(4):427–438, Oct 1978.

886. Holland RI. Fluoride inhibition of protein synthesis. *Cell Biol Int Rep* 3(9):701–705, Dec 1979.

887. Hurlbut WP, Ceccarelli B. Use of black widow spider venom to study the release of neurotransmitters. *Adv Cytopharmacol* 3:87–115, 1979.

888. Kelly RB, von Wedel RJ, Strong PN. Phospholipase-dependent and phospholipase-independent inhibition of transmitter release of beta-bungarotoxin. *Adv Cytopharmacol* 3:77–85, 1979.

889. Koch G, Koch F. The use of cytochalasins in studies on the molecular biology of virus-host cell interactions. *Front Biol* 46:475–498, 1978.

890. Lampe KF. Toxic fungi. *Annu Rev Pharmacol Toxicol* 19:85–104, 1979.

891. Lazdunski M, Balerna M, Chicheportiche R, Fosset M, Jacques Y, Lombet A, Romey G, Schweitz H. Interaction of neurotoxins with the selectivity filter and the gating system of the sodium channel. *Adv Cytopharmacol* 3:353–361, 1979.

892. Lee CY. Recent advances in chemistry and pharmacology of snake toxins. *Adv Cytopharmacol* 3:1–16, 1979.

893. Liehr H, Grun M. Endotoxins in liver disease. *Prog Liver Dis* 6:313–326, 1979.

894. Lorenz K. Ergot on cereal grains. *CRC Crit Rev Food Sci Nutr* 11(4):311–354, 1979.

895. Marsh N, Whaler B. The effects of snake venoms on the cardiovascular and haemostatic mechanisms. *Int J Biochem* 9(4):217–220, 1978.

896. McDonel JL. The molecular mode of action of Clostridium perfringens enterotoxin. *Am J Clin Nutr* 32(1):210–218, Jan 1979.

897. McGeer PL, McGeer EG. Use of the neurotoxic agents kainic acid and tetanus toxin in the extrapyramidal system. *Adv Cytopharmacol* 3:437–446, 1979.

898. McKinstry DM. Evidence of toxic saliva in some colubrid snakes of the United States. *Toxicon* 16(6):523–534, 1978.

899. Mongan PF. Tick toxicosis in North America. *J Fam Pract* 8(5):939–944, May 1979.

900. Morley BJ, Kemp GE, Salvaterra P. alpha-Bungarotoxin binding sites in the CNS. *Life Sci* 24(10):859–872, Mar 5, 1979.

901. Morrison DC, Ryan JL. Bacterial endotoxins and host immune responses. *Adv Immunol* 28:293–450, 1979.

902. Morrison DC, Ulevitch RJ. The effects of bacterial endotoxins on host mediation systems: a review. *Am J Pathol* 93(2):526–617, Nov 1978.

903. Moss J, Vaughan M. Activation of adenylate cyclase by choleragen. *Annu Rev Biochem* 48:581–600, 1979.

904. Neckers LM. Cholera toxin action in the central nervous system: effects on serotonin metabolism. *Adv Cytopharmacol* 3:447–453, 1979.

905. Newberne PM, Gross RL, Roe DA. Drug, toxin, and nutrient interactions. *Worl Rev Nutr Diet* 29:130–169, 1978.

906. O'Neill FJ. Control of nuclear division and chromosomal abnormalities in cytochalasin B-treated normal and transformed cells. *Front Biol* 46:217–255, 1978.

907. Pence HL. Stinging insect allergy. *Primary Care* 6(3):587–596, Sep 1979.

908. Rathmayer W. Sea anemone toxins: tools in the study of excitable membranes. *Adv Cytopharmacol* 3:335–344, 1979.

909. Reisman RE. Allergic reactions to insect stings. *South Med J* 71(2):208–209, 211, Feb 1978.

910. Richard JL, Thurston JR, Pier AC. Effects of mycotoxins on immunity. *Toxicon* (Suppl 1):801–817, 1978.

911. Richards KL, Douglas SD. Pathophysiological effects of Vibrio cholerae and enterotoxigenic Escherichia coli and their exotoxins on eucaryotic cells. *Microbiol Rev* 42(3):592–613, Sep 1978.

912. Rochat H, Bernard P, Couraud F. Scorpion toxins: chemistry and mode of action. *Adv Cytopharmacol* 3:325–334, 1979.

913. Rogolsky M. Nonenteric toxins of Staphylococcus aureus. *Microbiol Rev* 43(3):320–360, Sep 1979.

914. Schoental R. Mouldy grain and the aetiology of pellagra: the role of toxic metabolites of Fusarium. *Biochem Soc Trans* 8(1):147–150, Feb 1980.

915. Schroeder TE. Cytochalasin B, cytokinesis, and the contractile ring. *Front Biol* 46:91–112, 1978.

916. Simpson LL. Studies on the mechanism of action of botulinum toxin. *Adv Cytopharmacol* 3:27–34, 1979.

917. Tamm C. Chemistry and biosynthesis of cytochalasins. *Front Biol* 46:15–51, 1978.

918. Thesleff S, Lundh H. Mode of action of botulinum toxin and the effect of drug antagonists. *Adv Cytopharmacol* 3:35–43, 1979.

919. Thomas DD. Cytochalasin effects in plants and eukaryotic microbial systems. *Front Biol* 46:257–275, 1978.

920. Tilstone WJ, Winchester JF, Reavey PC. The use of pharmacokinetic principles in determining the effectiveness of removal of toxins from the blood. *Clin Pharmacokinet* 4(1):23–37, Jan-Feb 1979.

921. Ulbricht W. Kinetics of tetrodotoxin and saxitoxin action at the node of Ranvier. *Adv Cytopharmacol* 3:363–371, 1979.

922. Urbaschek B, Urbaschek R. The inflammatory response to endotoxins. *Bibl Anat* 17:74–104, 1979.

923. Walker RI. The contribution of intestinal endotoxin to mortality in hosts with compromised resistance: a review. *Exp Haematol* 6(2):172–184, Feb 1978.

924. Wickner RB. The killer double-stranded RNA plasmids of yeast. *Plasmid* 2(3):303–322, Jul 1979.

925. Wiegandt H. Toxin interactions with glycoconjugates. *Adv Cytopharmacol* 3:17–25, 1979.

926. Wieland, T, Faulstich H. Amatoxins, phallotoxins, phallolysin, and antamanide: the biologically active components of poisonous Amanita mushrooms. *CRC Crit Rev Biochem* 5(3):185–260, Dec 1978.

927. Yang CC. Chemistry and biochemistry of snake venom neurotoxins. *Toxicon* (Suppl 1):261–292, 1978.

Carcinogenesis, Mutagenesis, and Teratogenesis

928. Acrolein. *IARC Eval Carcinog Risk Chem Hum* 19:479–494, Feb 1979.

929. Acrylic acid, methyl acrylate, ethyl acrylate and polyacrylic acid. *IARC Monogr Eval Carcinog Risk Chem Hum* 19:47–71, Feb 1979.

930. Acrylonitrile, acrylic and modacrylic fibres, and acrylonitrile-butadiene-styrene and styrene-acylonitrile copolymers. *IARC Monogr Eval Carcinog Risk Chem Hum* 19:73–113, Feb 1979.

931. Adler ID. A review of the coordinated research effort on the comparison of test systems for the detection of mutagenic effects, sponsored by the E.E.C. *Mutat Res* 74(2):77–93, Apr 1980.

932. Ames BN. Identifying environmental chemicals causing mutations and cancer. *Science* 204(4393):587–593, May 11 1979.

933. Ashby J. Structural analysis as a means of predicting carcinogenic potential. *Br J Cancer* 37(6):904–923, Jun 1978.

934. Atal CK. Semisynthetic derivations of pyrrolizidine alkaloids of pharmacodynamic importance: a review. *Lloydia* 41(4):312–326, Jul-Aug 1978.

935. Bababunmi EA, Thabrew, I, Bassir O. Aflatoxin-induced coagulopathy in different nutritionally classified animal species. *World Rev Nutr Diet* 34:161–181, 1980.

936. Bababunmi EA, Uwaifo AO, Bassir O. Hepatocarcinogens in Nigerian foodstuffs. *World Rev Nutr Diet* 28:188–209, 1978.

937. Baden JM, Simmon VF. Mutagenic effects of inhalational anesthetics. *Mutat Res* 75(2):169–189, Mar 1980.

938. Barnes WS, Klekowski EJ Jr. Testing the environment for dispersed mutagens: use of plant bioconcentrators coupled with microbial mutagen assays. *Environ Health Perspect* 27:61–67, Dec 1978.

939. Baumann PA, Maitre L. Neurobiochemical aspects of maprotiline (Ludiomil) action. *J Int Med Res* 7(5):391–400, 1979.

940. Becci PJ, McDowell EM, Trump BF. The respiratory epithelium. VI. Histogenesis of lung tumors induced by benzo[a]pyrene-ferric oxide in the hamster. *JNCI* 61(2):607–618, Aug 1978.

941. Benedict WF, Jones PA. Mutagenic, clastogenic and oncogenic effects of 1-beta-D-arabinofuranosylcytosine. *Mutat Res* 65(1):1–20, Mar 1979.

942. Binns CH. Vinyl chloride: a review. *J Soc Occup Med* 29(4):134–141, Oct 1979.

943. Bolt HM. Pharmacokinetics of vinyl chloride. *Gen Pharmacol* 9(2):91–95, 1978.

944. Brambilla G, Cavanna M, Parodi S. Evaluation of DNA damage and repair in mammalian cells exposed to chemical carcinogens. Methods potentially useful as short term prescreening tests. *Pharmacol Res Commun* 10(8):693–717, Sep 1978.

945. Brash DE, Hart RW. DNA damage and repair in vivo. *J Environ Pathol Toxicol* 2(1):79–114, 1978.

946. Browne JC. Hormone administration during pregnancy and its effect on the offspring. *Contrib Gynecol Obstet* 5:56, 1979.

947. Brown WT. Human mutations affecting aging: a review. *Mech Ageing Dev* 9(3–4):325–336, Feb 1979.

948. Bueding E, Batzinger RP, Cha YN, Talalay P, Molineaux CJ. Protection from mutagenic effects of antischistosomal and other drugs. *Pharmacol Rev* 30(4):547–554, Dec 1978.

949. Callen DF. A review of the metabolism of xenobiotics by microorganisms with relation to short-term systems for environmental carcinogens. *Mutat Res* 55(3–4):153–163, 1978.

950. Caprolactam and nylon 6. *IARC Monogr Eval Carcinog Risk Chem Hum* 19:115–130, Feb 1979.

951. Carbon tetrachloride. *IARC Monogr Eval Carcinog Risk Chem Hum* 20:371–399, Oct 1979.

952. Chang CC, Trosko JE, Warren ST. In vitro assay for tumor promotors and anti-promotors. *J Environ Pathol Toxicol* 2(1):43–64, Sep-Oct 1978.

953. Chlordane. *IARC Monogr Eval Carcinog Risk Chem Hum* 20:45–65, Oct 1979.

954. Chloroform. *IARC Monogr Eval Carcinog Risk Chem Hum* 20:401–427, Oct 1979.

955. Cohen HS, Freedman ML, Goldstein BD. The problem of benzene in our environment: clinical and molecular considerations. *Am·J Med Sci* 275(2):124–36, Mar-Apr 1978.

956. Cohen MM, Shiloh Y. Genetic toxicology of lysergic acid diethylamide (LSD-25). *Mutat Res* 47(3–4):183–209, 1978.

957. Connor TH. The mutagenicity of trimethylphosphate. *Mutat Res* 65(2):121–31, 1979.

958. Constantin MJ. Utility of specific locus systems in higher plants to monitor for mutagens. *Environ Health Perspect* 27:69–75, Dec 1978.

959. Coombs MM. Chemical carcinogenesis: a view at the end of the first half-century. *J Pathol* 130(2):117–146, Feb 1980.

960. Daddona PE, Kelley WN. Adenosine deaminiase: characteristics of the normal and mutant forms of the human enzyme. *Ciba Found Symp* 68:177–91, 1978.

961. Daum SJ, Lemke JR. Mutational biosynthesis of new antibiotics. *Annu Rev Microbiol* 33:241–265, 1979.

962. Dean BJ. Genetic toxicology of benzene, toluene, xylenes and phenols. *Mutat Res* 47(2):75–97, 1978.

963. Diamond L, O'Brien TG, Rovera G. Tumor promoters: effects on proliferation and differentiation of cells in culture. *Life Sci* 23(20):1979–1988, Nov 13 1978.

964. 1,2-Dichloroethane. *IARC Monogr Eval Carcinog Risk Chem Hum* 20:429–448, Oct 1979.

965. Dichlorvos. *IARC Monogr Eval Carcinog Risk Chem Hum.* 20:97–127, Oct 1979.

966. Diethylstilboestrol and diethylstilboestrol dipropionate. *IARC Monogr Eval Carcinog Risk Chem Hum* 21:173–231, Dec 1979.

967. DiPaolo JA, Castro BC. In vitro carcinogenesis with cells in early passage. *Natl Cancer Inst Monogr* 48:245–257, May 1978.

968. Eisenbrand G. General review of approaches to nitrosamine analysis: derivative formation. *IARC Monogr Eval Carcinog Risk Chem Hum* 18:35–39, 1978.

969. Errera M. DNA repair and mutagenesis in bacterial systems and their implications in oncology. *Int J Radiat Oncol Biol Phys* 5(7):1077–1083, Jul 1979.

970. Ethinyloestradiol. *IARC Monogr Eval Carcinog Risk Chem Hum* 21:233–255, Dec 1979.

971. Ethylene and polyethylene. *IARC Monogr Eval Carcinog Risk Chem Hum* 19:157–186, Feb 1979.

972. Fishbein L. Overview of potential mutagenic problems posed by some pesticides and their trace impurities. *Environ Health Perspect* 27:125–131, Dec 1978.

973. Fishbein L. Overview of some aspects of occurrence, formation and analysis of nitrosamines. *Sci Total Environ* 13(2):157–188, Oct 1979.

974. Fishbein L. Potential halogenated industrial carcinogenic and mutagenic chemicals. I. Halogenated unsaturated hydrocarbons. *Sci Total Environ* 11(2):111–161, Mar 1979.

975. Fishbein L. Potential halogenated industrial carcinogenic and mutagenic chemicals. II. Halogenated saturated hydrocarbons. *Sci Total Environ* 11(2):163–195, Mar 1979.

976. Fishbein L. Potential halogenated industrial carcinogenic and mutagenic chemicals. III. Alkane halides, alkanols and ethers. *Sci Total Environ* 11(3):223–257, Apr 1979.

977. Fishbein L. Potential halogenated industrial carcinogenic and mutagenic chemicals. IV. Halogenated aryl derivatives. *Sci Total Environ* 11(3):259–278, Apr 1979.

978. Forni A. Chromosome changes and benzene exposure: a review. *Rev Environ Health* 3(1):5–17, 1979.

979. Forsberg JG. Physiological mechanisms of diethylstilbestrol organotropic carcinogenesis. *Arch Toxicol [Suppl]* 2:263–274, 1979.

980. Fox M, Scott D. The genetic toxicology of nitrogen and sulphur mustard. *Mutat Res* 75(2):131–168, Mar 1980.

981. Francois J, DeBie S, Leuven MT. The Costenbader Memorial Lecture. Genesis and genetics of retinoblastoma. *J. Pediatr Ophthalmol Strabismus* 16(2):85–100, Mar-Apr 1979.

982. Freeling M. Maize Adhl as a monitor of environmental mutagens. *Environ Health Perspect* 27:91–97, Dec 1978.

983. Friis RR. Temperature-sensitive mutants of avian RNA tumor viruses: a review. *Curr Top Microbiol Immunol* 79:261–293, 1978.

984. Geelen JA. Hypervitaminosis A induced teratogenesis. *CRC Crit Rev Toxicol* 6(4):351–375, Nov 1979.

985. General remarks on sex hormones. *IARC Monogr Eval Carcinog Risk Chem Hum* 21:33–82, Dec 1979.

986. Goldfarb RH, Quigley JP. Synergistic effect of tumor virus transformation and tumor promoter treatment on the production of plasminogen activator by chick embryo fibroblasts. *Cancer Res* 38(12):4601–4609, Dec 1978.

987. Glubovskaya IN. Genetic control of meiosis. *Int Rev Cytol* 58:247–290, 1979.

988. Gough TA. Determination of N-nitroso compounds by mass spectrometry. *Analyst* 103(1229):785–806, Aug 1978.

989. Gough TA. General review of approaches to nitrosamine analysis: mass spectrometric techniques. *IARC Sci Publ* 18:29–34, 1978.

990. Grigg GW. Genetic effects of coumarins. *Mutat Res* 47(3–4):161–181, 1978.

991. Gronow M. Nuclear proteins and chemical carcinogenesis. *Chem Biol Interact* 29(1):1–30, Jan 1980.

992. Gurtoo HL, Dahms R, Vaught JB. Metabolism of a prototype mycotoxin, aflatoxin B1, and its genetic regulation. *Mycopathologis* 65(1–3):13 Dec 18 1978.

993. Haley TJ. Chloroprene (2-chloro-1,3 butadiene)—what is the evidence for its carcinogenicity? *Clin Toxicol* 13(2):153–170.

994. Hall JG, Pauli RM, Wilson KM. Maternal and fetal sequelae of anticoagulation during pregnancy. *Am J Med* 68(1):122–140, Jan 1980.

995. Hancock RL, Hancock CD. Theoretical mechanisms for synthesis of carcinogen-induced embryonic proteins: III. The tRNA methylases; methylation mechanism and function. *Med Hypotheses* 4(5):497–515, Sep-Oct 1978.

996. Hankin JH, Rawling V. Diet and breast cancer: a review. *Am J Clin Nutr* 31(11):2005–2016, Nov 1978.

997. Harshbarger JC. Role of the registry of tumors in lower animals in the study of environmental carcinogenesis in aquatic animals. *Ann NY Acad Sci* 298:280–289, Sep 29 1978.

998. Hart RW, Hall KY, Daniel FB. DNA repair and mutagenesis in mammalian cells. *Photochem Photobiol* 28(2):131–155, Aug 1978.

999. Hayes AW. Biological activities of mycotoxins. *Mycopathologia* 65(1–3):29–41, Dec 18 1978.

1000. Hemminki, Sorsa M, Vainio H. Genetic risks caused by occupational chemicals. Use of experimental methods and occupational risk group monitoring in the detection of environmental chemicals causing mutations, cancer and malformations. *Scand J Work Environ Health* 5(4):307–327, Dec 1979.

1001. Heppleston AG, Silica and asbestos: contrasts in tissue response. *Ann NY Acad Sci* 330:725–744, 1979.

1002. Heptachlor and heptachlor epoxide. *IARC Monogr Eval Carcinog Risk Chem Hum* 20:129–154, Oct 1979.

1003. Hexachlorobenzene. *IARC Monogr Eval Carcinog Risk Chem Hum* 20:155–178, Oct 1979.

1004. Hexachlorcyclohexane (technical HCH and lindane). *IARC Monogr Eval Carcinog Risk Chem Hum* 20:195–239, Oct 1979.

1005. Hexachlorophene. *IARC Monogr Eval Carcinog Risk Chem Hum* 20:241–257, Oct 1979.

1006. Hickey RJ, Clelland RC, Bowers EJ. Essential hormones as carcinogenic hazards. *JOM* 21(4):265–268, Apr 1979.

1007. Higginson J, Muir CS. Environmental carcinogenesis: misconceptions and limiations to cancer control. *JNCI* 63(6):1291–1298, Dec 1979.

1008. Hill MJ. Role of bacteria in human carcinogenesis. *J Hum Nutr* 33(6):416–426, Dec 1979.

1009. Hoffman D, Wynder EL. Identification and reduction of carcinogens in the respiratory environment. *Zentralbl Bakteriol [Orig B]* (2–3):113–135, Mar 1978.

1010. Hoffman GR. Genetic effects of dimethyl sulfate, diethyl sulfate, and related compounds. *Mutat Res* 75(1):63–129, Jan 1980.

1011. Hollstein M. McCann J. Angelosanto FA, Nichols WW. Short-term tests for carcinogens and mutagens. *Mutat Res* 65(3):133–226, Sep 1979.

1012. Homburger F. Chemical carcinogenesis in Syrian hamsters: a review (through 1976). *Prog Exp Tumor Res* 23:100–179, 1979.

1013. Howard FM, Hill JM. Drugs in pregnancy. *Obstet Gynecol Surv* 34(9):643–653, Sep 1979.

1014. Huxtable RJ. New aspects of the toxicology and pharmacology of pyrrolizidine alkaloids. *Gen Pharmacol* 10(3):159–167, 1979.

1015. Izard C, Libermann C. Acrolein. *Mutat Res* 47(2):115–138, 1978.

1016. Jacobs M. A critical review: will the Ames Salmonella assay system be used as a screen for presumptive carcinogens? *J Environ Pathol Toxicol* 2(4):1205–1215, Mar-Apr 1979.

1017. Jurgelski W Jr, Hudson P, Falk HL. Tissue differentiation and susceptibility to embryonal tumor induction by ethylnitrosourea in the opossum. *Natl Cancer Inst Monogr* 51:123–158, May 1979.

1018. Kadlubar FF, Miller JA, Miller EC. Guanyl 06-arylamination and 06-arylation of DNA by the carcinogen N-hydroxy-1-naphthylamine. *Cancer Res* 38(11 Part 1):3628–3638, Nov 1978.

1019. Kannerstien M, Churg J, McCaughey WT. Asbestos and mesothelioma: a review. *Pathol Ann* 13 (Part 1):81–129, 1978.

1020. Kimball RF. The relation of repair phenomena to mutation induction in the bacteria. *Mutat Res* 55(2):85–120, 1978.

1021. Klein J. H-2 mutations: their genetics and effect on immune functions. *Adv Immunol* 26:55–146, 1978.

1022. Kurman RJ. Abnormalities of the genital tract following stilbestrol exposure in utero. *Recent Results Cancer Res* 66:161–174, 1979.

1023. LaMont JT, O'Gorman TA. Experimental colon cancer. *Gastroenterology* 75(6):1157–1169, Dec 1978.

1024. Lee IP, Dixon RL. Mutagenicity, carcinogenicity and teratogenicity of procarbazine. *Mutat Res* 55(1):1–14, 1978.

1025. Leonard A, Lauwerys RR. Carcinogenicity, teratogenicity and mutagenicity of arsenic. *Mutat Res* 75(1):49–62, Jan 1980.

1026. Litwin JA. Histochemistry and cytochemistry of 3,3'-diaminobenzidine: a review. *Folia Histochem Cytochem (Krakow)* 17(1):3–28, 1979.

1027. Lutz WK. In vivo covalent binding of organic chemicals to DNA as a quantitative indicator in the process of chemical carcinogenesis. *Mutat Res* 65(4):289–356, Dec 1979.

1028. Melzer MS. Critique of "carcinogen-induced repair DNA synthesis". *Cell Biol Int Rep* 3(7):559–571, Oct 1979.

1029. Melzer MS. Paradox of carcinogens as cell destroyers and cell stimulators. A biochemical hypothesis. *Eur J Cancer* 16(1):15–22, Jan 1980.

1030. Mestranol. *IARC Monogr Eval Carcinog Risk Chem Hum* 21:257–278, Dec 1979.

1031. Methoxychlor. *IARC Monogr Eval Carcinog Risk Chem Hum* 20:259–281, Oct 1979.

1032. Methyl metacrylate and polymethyl methacrylate. *IARC Monogr Eval Carcinog Risk Chem Hum* 19:187–211, Feb 1979.

1033. Metzler M, McLachlan JA. Diethylstilbestrol metabolic transformation in relation to organ specific tumor manifestation. *Arch Toxicol [Suppl]* 2:275–280, 1979.

1034. Miller AB. Asbestos fibre dust and gastro-intestinal malignancies. Review of literature with regard to a cause/effect relationship. *J Chronic Dis* 31(1):23–33, Jan 1978.

1035. Miller EC, Miller JA. Milestones in chemical carcinogenesis. *Semin Oncol* 6(4):445-460, Dec 1979.

1036. Miller EC. Some current perspectives on chemical carcinogenesis in humans and experimental animals: Presidential address. *Cancer Res* 38(6):1479-1496, Jun 1978.

1037. Miller K. The effects of asbestos on macrophages. *CRC Crit Rev Toxicol* 5(4):319-354, Sep 1978.

1038. Miller RW. Environmental causes of cancer in childhood. *Adv Pediatr* 25:97-119.

1039. Mirex. *IARC Monogr Eval Carcinog Risk Chem Hum* 20:283-301, Oct 1979.

1040. Montesano R. The use of mutagenicity tests in screening chemical carcinogens. *Prog Biochem Pharmacol* 14:157-162, 1978.

1041. Montouris GD, Fenichel GM, McLain LW Jr. The pregnant epileptic: a review and recommendations. *Arch Neurol* 36(10):601-603, Oct 1979.

1042. Moore MR, Meredith PA. The carcinogenicity of lead. *Arch Toxicol* 42(2):87-94, Jun 1979.

1043. Mulcahy DL, Johnson CM. Self-incompatibility systems as bioassays for mutagens. *Environ Health Perspect* 27:85-90, Dec 1978.

1044. Munthe-Kaas AC. Kupffer cell suspensions and cultures as a tool in experimental carcinogenesis. *J Toxicol Environ Health* 5(2-3):565-73, Mar-May 1979.

1045. Murthy MS. Induction of gene conversion in diploid yeast by chemicals: correlation with mutagenic action and its relevance in genotoxicity screening. *Mutat Res* 64(1):1-17, Feb 1979.

1046. Nagao M, Sugimura T, Matsushima T. Environmental mutagens and carcinogens. *Ann Rev Genet* 12:117-159, 1978.

1047. Nassim A, Brychcy T. Genetic effects of acridine compounds. *Mutat Res* 65(4):261-288, Dec 1979.

1048. Nebert DW, Jensen NM. The Ah locus: genetic regulation of the metabolism of carcinogens, drugs, and other environmental chemicals by cytochrome P-450-mediated monooxygenases. *CRC Crit Rev Biochem* 6(4):401-437, 1979.

1049. Nilan RA. Potential of plant genetic systems for monitoring and screening mutagens. *Environ Health Perspect* 27:181-196, Dec 1978.

1050. N-nitrosodiethylamine. *IARC Monogr Eval Carcinog Risk Chem Man* 17:83-124, May 1978.

1051. N-nitrosodiemethylamine. *IARC Monogr Eval Carcinog Risk Chem Man* 17:125-175, May 1978.

1052. N-Nitroso-N-ethylurea. *IARC Monogr Eval Carcinog Risk Chem Man* 17:191–215, May 1978.

1053. N-nitroso-N-methylurea. *IARC Monogr Eval Carcinog Risk Chem Man* 17:227–255, May 1978.

1054. N-nitrosopyrrolidine. *IARC Monogr Eval Carcinog Risk Chem Man* 17:313–326, May 1978.

1055. Norethisterone and norethisterone acetate. *IARC Monogr Eval Carcinog Risk Chem Hum* 21:441–460, Dec 1979.

1056. Norethynodrel. *IARC Monogr Eval Carcinog Risk Chem Hum* 21:461–477, Dec 1979.

1057. Oakley GP Jr. Drug influences on malformations. *Clin Perinatol* 6(2):403–414, Sep 1979.

1058. Obe G, Ristow H. Mutagenic, cancerogenic and teratogenic effects of alcohol. *Mutat Res* 65(4):229–259, Dec 1979.

1059. Obe G, Beek B. Trenimon: biochemical, physiological and genetic effects on cells and organisms. *Mutat Res* 65(1):21–70, Mar 1979.

1060. Oestrogens and progestins in relation to human cancer. *IARC Monogr Eval Carcinog Risk Chem Hum* 21:83–129, Dec 1979.

1061. Olajos EJ, Coulston F. Comparative toxicology of N-nitroso compounds and their carcinogenic potential to man. *Ecotoxicol Environ Safety* 2(3-4):317–367, Dec 1978.

1062. Ong TM. Genetic activities of hycanthone and some other antischistosomal drugs. *Mutat Res* 55(1):43–70, 1978.

1063. Pentachlorophenol. *IARC Monogr Eval Carcinog Risk Chem Hum* 20:303–325, Oct 1979.

1064. Plewa MJ. Activation of chemicals into mutagens by green plants: a preliminary discussion. *Environ Health Perspect* 27:45–50, Dec 1978.

1065. Poirier LA, Weisburger EK. Selection of carcinogens and related compounds tested for mutagenic activity. *JNCI* 62(4):833–840, Apr 1979.

1066. Polybrominated biphenyls. *IARC Monog Eval Carcinog Risk Chem Hum* 18:104–124, Oct 1978.

1067. Polychlorinated biphenyls. *IARC Monogr Eval Carcinog Risk Chem Hum* 18:41–103, Oct 1978.

1068. Preussmann R. Toxicological aspects of food safety—carcinogenicity and mutagenecity. *Arch Toxicol [Suppl]* (1):69–84, 1978.

1069. Progesterone. *IARC Monogr Eval Carcinog Risk Chem Hum* 21:491–515, Dec 1979.

1070. Purchase IF. Procedures for screening chemicals for carcinogenicity. *Br J Ind Med* 37(1):1–10, Feb 1980.

1071. Purnell DM. Virulence genetics of Aspergillus nidulans Eidam: a review. *Mycopathologia* 65(1-3):177-182, Dec 18 1978.

1072. Ray VA. Application of microbial and mammalian cells to the assessment of mutagenicity. *Pharmacol Rev* 30(4):537-546, Dec 1978.

1073. Reuber MD. Carcinogenicity of endrin. *Sci Total Environ* 72(2):101-135, Jun 1979.

1074. Reuber MD. The carcinogenicity of kepone. *J. Environ Pathol Toxicol* 2(3):671-686, Jan-Feb 1979.

1075. Reuber MD. Carcinogenicity of kepone. *J. Toxicol Environ Health* 4(5-6):895-911, Sep-Nov 1978.

1076. Reuber MD. Carcinogenicity of lindane. *Environ Res* 19(2):460-481, Aug 1979.

1077. Reuber MD. Carcinogenicity of saccharin. *Environ Health Perspect* 25:173-200, Aug 1978.

1078. Reuber MD. Carcinogenicity of toxaphene: a review. *J Toxicol Envion Health* 5(4):729-748, Jul 1979.

1079. Rinkus SJ, Legator MS. Chemical characterization of 465 known or suspected carcinogens and their correlation with mutagenic activity in the Salmonella typhimurium system. *Cancer Res* 39(9):3289-3318, Sep 1979.

1080. Roboz J. Mass spectrometry in cancer research. *Adv Cancer Res* 27:201-267, 1978.

1081. Rodighiero G. The problem of the carcinogenic risk by furocoumarins. *Prog Biochem Pharmacol* 14:94-103, 1978.

1082. Ronen A. 2-Aminopurine. *Mutat Res* 75(1):1-47, Jan 1980.

1083. Sandor S. The prenatal noxious effect of ethanol. *Morphol Embryol (Bucur)* 25(3):211-223, Jul-Sep 1979.

1084. Schlaet AP. Interspecific comparison of ethyl methanesulfonate-methanesulfonate-induced mutation rates in relation to genome size. *Mutat Res* 49(3):313-340, Mar 1978.

1085. Schenker MB. Diesel exhaust—an occupational carcinogen? *JOM* 22(1):41-46, Jan 1980.

1086. Schmahl D, Habs M. Experimental carcinogenesis of antitumour drugs. *Cancer Treat Rev* 5(4):175-184, Dec 1978.

1087. Scribner JD, Suss R. Tumor initiation and promotion. *Int Rev Exp Pathol* 18:137-198, 1978.

1088. Selkirk JK. Analysis of benzo[a]pyrene metabolism by high-pressure liquid chromatography. *Adv Chromatogr* 16:1-36, 1978.

1089. Sell S. AFP as a marker for liver cell injury: differentiation of tumor growth, hepatotoxicity, and carcinogenesis. *UCLA Forum Med Sci* 20:51–58, 1978.

1090. Sen NP. General review of approaches to nitrosamine analysis: final chromatography and detection. *IARC Sci Publ* 18:21–27, 1978.

1091. Shabad LM. Circulation of carcinogenic polycyclic aromatic hydrocarbons in the human environment and cancer prevention. *JNCI* 64(3):405–410, Mar 1980.

1092. Simchen G. Cell cycle mutants. *Ann Rev Genet* 12:161–191, 1978.

1093. Singer B. N-nitroso alkylating agents: formation and persistence of alkyl derivatives in mammalian nucleic acids as contributing factors in carcinogenesis. *JNCI* 62(6):1329–1339, Jun 1979.

1094. Sivak A. Overview and status of in vitro transformation. *J Assoc Off Anal Chem* 62(4):889–899, Jul 1979.

1095. Slater TF. Biochemical studies of transient intermediates in relation to chemical carcinogenesis. *Ciba Found Symp* 67:301–328, 1978.

1096. Smith KC. Multiple pathways of DNA repair and their possible roles in mutagenesis. *Natl Cancer Inst Mongr* 50:107–114, Dec 1978.

1097. Smith KC. Multiple pathways of DNA repair in bacteria and their roles in mutagenesis. *Photochem Photobiol* 28(2):121–129, Aug 1978.

1098. Smythies JR. On the relation between chemical structure and function in certain tumor promoters and antitumor agents. *Prog Drug Res* 23:63–96, 1979.

1099. Sternberg SS. The carcinogenesis, mutagenisis and teratogenesis of insecticides. Review of studies in animals and man. *Pharmacol Ther* 6(1):147–166, 1979.

1100. Stich HF, Whiting RF, Wei L, San RH. DNA fragmentation and DNA repair of mammalian cells as an indicator for the complex interactions between carcinogens and modulating factors. *Pharmacol Rev* 30(4):493–499, Dec 1978.

1101. Stumpf DA, Frost M. Seizures, anticonvulsants, and pregnancy. *Am J Dis Child* 132(8):746–748, Aug 1978.

1102. Styrene, polystyrene and styrene-butadiene copolymers. *IARC Monogr Eval Carcinog Risk Chem Hum* 19:231–274, Feb 1979.

1103. Sugimura T, Nagao M. Mutagenic factors in cooked foods. *CRC Crit Rev Toxicol* 6(3):189–209, Aug 1979.

1104. Sula J. Experimental data concerning the question of the synergic action of the influenza virus and of some chemical carcinogens in the pathogenesis of lung cancer. *Neoplasma* 26(1):17–22, 1979.

1105. Sunderman FW Jr. Carcinogenic effects of metals. *Fed Proc* 37(1):40–46, Jan 1978.

1106. Telling GM. General review of approaches to nitrosamine analysis: extraction and clean-up methods. *IARC Sci Publ* 18:15-20, 1978.

1007. Testosterone, testosterone oenanthate and testosterone propionate. *IARC Monogr Eval Carcinog Risk Chem Hum* 21:519-547, Dec 1979.

1108. Tetrachloroethylene. *IARC Monogr Eval Carcinog Risk Chem Hum* 20:491-514, Oct 1979.

1109. Tetrafluoroethylene and polytetrafluoroethylene. *IARC Monogr Eval Carcinog Risk Chem Hum* 19:285-301, Feb 1979.

1110. 2,4- and 2,6-toluene diisocyanates, 1,5-naphthalene diisocyanate, 4,4-methylenediphenyl diisocyanate and polymethylene polyphenyl isocyanate and flexible and rigid polyurethane foams. *IARC Monogr Eval Carcinog Risk Chem Hum* 19:303-340, Feb 1979.

1111. Tomatis L, Agthe C, Bartsch H, Huff J, Montesano R, Saracci R, Walker E, Wilbourn J. Evaluation of the carcinogenicity of chemicals: a review of the Monograph Program of the International Agency for Research on Cancer (1971-1977). *Cancer Res* 38(4):877-885, Apr 1978.

1112. Tomatis L. The predictive value of rodent carcinogenicity tests in the evaluation of human risks. *Ann Rev Pharmacol Toxicol* 19:511-520, 1979.

1113. Tomatis L. Prenatal exposure to chemical carcinogens and its effect on subsequent generations. *Natl Cancer Inst Monogr* 51:159-184, May 1979.

1114. Toxaphene (polychlorinated camphenes). *IARC Monogr Eval Carcinog Risk Chem Hum* 20:327-348, Oct 1979.

1115. 1,1,1-Trichloroethane. *IARC Monogr Eval Carcinog Risk Chem Hum* 20:515-531, Oct 1979.

1116. Trichloroethylene. *IARC Monogr Eval Carinog Risk Chem Hum* 20:545-572, Oct 1979.

1117. Trosko JE, Chang CC. Environmental carcinogenesis: an integrative model. *Q Rev Biol* 53(2):115-141, Jun 1978.

1118. Trosko JE, Chang C. Genes, pollutants and human diseases. *Q Rev Biophys* 11(4):603-627, Nov 1978.

1119. Trosko JE, Chang CC. Relationship between mutagenesis and carcinogenesis. *Photochem Photobiol* 28(2):157-168, Aug 1978.

1120. Vainio H. Vinyl chloride and vinyl benzene (styrene)-metabolism, mutagenicity and carcinogenicity. *Chem Biol Interact* 22(1):117-124, Jul 1978.

1121. VanBlerk GA, Majerus TC, Myers RA. Teratogenic potential of some psychopharmacologic drugs: a brief review. *Int J Gynaecol Obstet* 17(4):399-402, Jan-Feb 1980.

1122. Vesselinovitch SD, Rao KV, Mihailovich N. Neoplastic response of mouse tissues during perinatal age periods and its significance in chemical carcinogenesis. *Natl Cancer Inst Monogr* 51:239–250, May 1979.

1123. Vig BK. Mutagenic effects of some anticancer antibiotics. *Cancer Chemother Pharmacol* 3(3):143–160, 1979.

1124. Vig BK, Lewis R. Genetic toxicology of bleomycin. *Mutat Res* 55(2):121–145, 1978.

1125. Vinyl bromide. *IARC Monogr Eval Carcinog Risk Chem Hum* 19:367–375, Feb 1979.

1126. Vinyl chloride, polyvinyl chloride and vinyl chloride-vinyl acetate copolymers. *IARC Monogr Eval Carcinog Risk Chem Hum* 19:377–438, Feb 1979.

1127. Vinylidene chloride and vinylidene chloride-vinyl chloride copolymers. *IARC Monogr Eval Carcinog Risk Chem Hum* 19:439–459, Feb 1979.

1128. N-vinyl-2-pyrrolidone and polyvinyl pyrrolidone. *IARC Monogr Eval Monogr Eval Carcinog Risk Chem Hum* 19:461–477, Feb 1979.

1129. Wassom JS, Huff JE, Loprieno N. A review of the genetic toxicology of chlorinated dibenzo-p-dioxins. *Mutat Res* 47(3–4):141–160, 1978.

1130. Wattenberg LW. Inhibition of chemical carcinogenesis. *J Natl Cancer Inst* 60(1):11–18, Jan 1978.

1131. Wattenberg LW. Inhibitors of chemical carcinogenesis. *Adv Cancer Res* 26:197–226, 1978.

1132. Wechsler W, Rice JM, Vesselinovitch SD. Transplacental and neonatal induction of neurogenic tumors in mice: comparison with related species and with human pediatric neoplasms. *Natl Cancer Inst Monogr* 51:219–226, May 1979.

1133. Weinstein IB, Lee LS, Fisher PB, Mufson A, Yamasaki H. Action of phorbol esters in cell culture: mimicry of transformation, altered differentiation, and effects on cell membranes. *J. Supramol Struct* 12(2):195–208, 1979.

1134. Weisburger EK. Mechanisms of chemical carcinogenesis. *Annu Rev Pharmacol Toxicol* 18:395–415, 1978.

1135. Weisburger JH. Environmental cancer: on the causes of the main human cancers. *Tex Rep Biol Med* 37:1–20, 1978.

1136. Wildenberg J. An assessment of experimental carcinogen-detecting systems with special reference to inorganic arsenicals. *Environ Res* 16(1–3):139–152, Jul 1978.

1137. Williams GM. Review of in vitro test systems using DNA damage and repair for screening of chemical carcinogens. *J Assoc Off Anal Chem* 62(4):857–863, Jul 1979.

1138. Wilson JG. Review of in vitro systems with potential for use in teratogenicity screening. *J Environ Pathol Toxicol* 2(1):149–167, Sep-Oct 1978.

1139. Wolman SR. Mutational consequences of exposure to ethylene oxide. *J Environ Pathol Toxicol* 2(6):1289–1303, Jul-Aug 1979.

1140. Wright AS. The role of metabolism in chemical mutagenesis and chemical carcinogenesis. *Mutat Res* 75(2):215–41, Mar 1980.

1141. Zachowski A, Lelievre L, Geny B, Charlamagne D, Aubry J, Paraf A. Cell lines with altered membrane structures for comprehensive studies of cancer cells. *Prog Exp Tumor Res* 22:28–78, 1978.

1142. Zbinden G, Bachmann E, Holderegger C. Model systems for cardiotoxic effects of anthracyclines. *Antibiot Chemother* 23:255–270, 1978.

1143. Zenz C. Benzene-attempts to establish a lower exposure standard in the United States: a review. *Scand J Work Environ Health* 4(2):103–113, Jun 1978.

Cosmetics

1144. Ali AR, Smales OR, Aslam M. Surma and lead poisoning. *Br Med J* 2(6142):915–916, Sep 30 1978.

1145. 4-amino-2-nitrophenol. *IARC Monogr Eval Carcinog Risk Chem Man* 16:43–49, Jan 1978.

1146. Andersen KE. Contact allergy to toothpaste flavors. *Contact Dermatitis* 4(4):195–198, Aug 1978.

1147. Aune T, Nelson SD, Dybing E. Mutagenicity and irreversible binding of the hepatocarcinogen, 2,4-diaminotoluene. *Chem Biol Interact* 25(1):23–33, Apr 1979.

1148. Bernstein ML. Oral mucosal white lesions associated with excessive use of Listerine mouthwash. Report of two cases. *Oral Surg* 46(6):781–785, Dec 1978.

1149. Borum P, Holten A, Loekkegaard N. Depression of nasal mucociliary transport by an aerosol hair-spray. *Scand J Respir Dis* 60(5):253–259, Oct 1979.

1150. Burger PM, Simons JW. Mutagenicity and carcinogenicity of 8-MOP/UVA in cell culture. *Bull Cancer* (Paris) 65(3):281–282, 1978.

1151. Burnett CM, Corbett JF, Lanman BM. Hair dyes and aplastic anemia. *Drug Chem Toxicol* 1(1):45–61, 1977–78.

1152. Cinnamyl anthranilate. *IARC Monogr Eval Carcinog Risk Chem Man* 16:287–291, Jan 1978.

1153. Cohen BM. Respiratory responses to one year of daily use of cosmetic hair spray. *Lung* 155(4):309–320, Dec 15 1978.

1154. Cronin E. Immediate-type hypersensitivity to henna. *Contact Dermatitis* 5(3):198–199, May 1979.

1155. Cronin E, Kullavanijaya P. Hand dermatitis in hairdressers. *Acta Derm Venereol* (Suppl) (Stockholm) 59(85):47–50, 1979.

1156. Davies MG, Hodgson GA, Evans E. Contact dermatitis from an ostomy deodorant. *Contact Dermatitis* 4(1):11–13, Feb 1978.

1157. 2,4-diaminoanisole (sulphate). *IARC Monogr Eval Carcinog Risk Chem Man* 16:51–62, Jan 1978.

1158. 1,2-diamino-4-nitrobenzene. *IARC Monogr Eval Carcinog Risk Chem Man* 16:73–82, Jan 1978.

1159. 1,4-diamino-2-nitrobenzene. *IARC Monogr Eval Carcinog Risk Chem Man* 16:73–82, Jan 1978.

1160. 2,5-diaminotoluene (sulphate). *IARC Monogr Eval Carcinog Risk Chem Man* 16:97–109, Jan 1978.

1161. Dogliotti M, Leibowitz M. Granulomatous ochronosis: a cosmetic-induced skin disorder in Blacks. *S Afr Med* 56(19):757–760, Nov 3 1979.

1162. Dooms-Goossens A, Degreef H, Luytens E. Dihydroabietyl alcohol (Abitol): a sensitizer in mascara. *Contact Dermatitis* 5(6):350–353, Dec 1979.

1163. Epstein WL, Taylor MK. Experimental sensitization to paraphenylene-diamine and paratoluenediamine in man. *Acta Derm Venereol* (Suppl) (Stockholm) 59(85):55–57, 1979.

1164. Farber EM. Psoralen and ultraviolet A (PUVA): a critique. *J Am Acad Dermatol* 2(4):342–344, Apr 1980.

1165. Findlay GH, de Beer HA. Chronic hydroquinone poisoning of the skin from skin-lightening cosmetics. A South African epidemic of ochronosis of the face in dark-skinned individuals. *S Afr Med J* 57(6):187–190, Feb 9 1980.

1166. Fisher AA. Dermatitis due to formaldehyde-releasing agents in cosmetics and medicaments. *Cutis* 22(6):655, 658, 662, Dec 1978.

1167. Formicola AJ, Deasy MJ, Johnson DH, Howe EE. Tooth staining effects of an alexidine mouthwash. *J Periodontol* 50(4):207–211, Apr 1979.

1168. Heywood R, Sortwell RJ, Noel PR, Street AE, Prentice DE, Roe FJ, Wadsworth PF, Worden AN, Van Abbe NJ. Safety evaluation of toothpaste containing chloroform. III. Long term study in beagle dogs. *J Environ Pathol Toxicol* 2(3):835–851, Jan-Feb 1979.

1169. Hennekens CH, Speizer FE, Rosner B, Bain CJ, Belanger C, Peto R. Use of permanent hair dyes and cancer among registered nurses. *Lancet* 1(8131):1390–1393, Jun 30 1979.

1170. Hoffman TE, Adams RM. Contact dermatitis to benzoin in greasepaint makeup. *Contact Dermatitis* 4(6):379-380, Dec 1978.

1171. IARC monographs on the evaluation of the carcinogenic risk of chemicals to man: general remarks on the substances considered. *IARC Mongr Carcinog Risk Chem Man* 16:25-37, Jan 1978.

1172. Incidence of allergic reactions to coal tar dyes in patients with cosmetic dermatitis. *J Dermatol* (Tokyo) 5(6):291-295, Dec 1978.

1173. Johnson SP. Hair dyes and the chromosomes. *Food Cosmet Toxicol* 17(3):301-303, Jun 1979.

1174. Lerman S, Megaw J, Willis I. Potential ocular complications from PUVA therapy and their prevention. *J Invest Dermatol* 74(4):197-199, Apr 1980.

1175. Light green SF. *IARC Mongr Eval Carcinog Risk Chem Man* 16:209-220, Jan 1978.

1176. Longo DL, Young RC. Cosmetic talc and ovarian cancer. *Lancet* 2(8138):349-351, Aug 18 1979.

1177. Mathias CG, Chappler RR, Maibach HI. Contact urticaria from cinnamic aldehyde. *Arch Dermatol* 116(1):74-76, Jan 1980.

1178. Mathias CG, Cram D, Ragsdale J, Maibach HI. Contact dermatitis caused by spouse's perfume and cologne. *Can Med Assoc J* 119(3):257-258, Aug 12 1978.

1179. Marzulli FN, Green S, Maibach HI. Hair dye toxicity: a review. *J Environ Pathol Toxicol* 1(4):509-530, Mar-Apr 1978.

1180. Menkart J. An analysis of adverse reactions to cosmetics. *Cutis* 24(6):599, 662 Dec 1979.

1181. Menkart J. Cosmetic ingredient labelling. *Cutis* 24(1):35, Jul 1979.

1182. Menkart J. Hair coloring: a case study in risk assessment. *Cutis* 22(6):670, 693, 724 Dec 1978.

1183. Meta-phenylenediamine (hydrochloride). *IARC Monogr Eval Carcinog Risk Chem Man* 16:111-124, Jan 1978.

1184. Murphy SB, Jackson WB, Pare JA. Talc retinopathy. *Can J Ophthalmol* 13(3):152-156, Jul 1978.

1185. Nasca PC, Lawrence CE, Greenwald P, Chorost S, Arbuckle JT, Paulson A. *JNCI* 64(1):23-28, Jan 1980.

1186. Palmer AK, Street AE, Roe FJ, Worden AN, van Abbe NJ. Safety evaluation of toothpaste containing chloroform. II. Long term studies in rats. *J Environ Pathol Toxicol* 2(3):821-833, Jan-Feb 1979.

1187. Para-phenylenediamine (hydrochloride). *IARC Monogr Eval Carcinog Risk Chem Man* 16:125-142, Jan 1978.

1188. Prival MJ, Mitchell VD, Gomez YP. Mutagenicity of a new hair dye ingredient: 4-ethoxy-m-phenylenediamine. *Science* 207(4433):907–908, Feb 15 1980.

1189. Raugi GJ, Storrs FJ, Larsen WG. Photoallergic contact dermatitis to men's perfumes. *Contact Dermatitis* 5(4):251–260, Jul 1979.

1190. Reid FR, Wood TO. Pseudomonas corneal ulcer: the causative role of contaminated eye cosmetics. *Arch Ophthalmol* 97(9):1640–1641, Sep 1979.

1191. Rhodamine B. *IARC Monogr Carcinog Risk Chem Man* 16:221–231, Jan 1978.

1192. Rhodamine 6B. *IARC Monogr Eval Carcinog Risk Chem Man* 16:233–239, Jan 1978.

1193. Roe FJ, Palmer AK, Worden AN, van Abbe NJ. Safety evaluation of toothpaste containing chloroform. I. Long-term studies in mice. *J Environ Pathol Toxicol* 2(3):799–819, Jan-Feb 1979.

1194. Schlueter DP, Soto RJ, Baretta ED, Herrmann AA, Ostrander LE, Stewart RD. Airway response to hair spray in normal subjects and subjects with hyperreactive airways. *Chest* 75(5):544–548, May 1979.

1195. Sharp DW. The sensitization potential of some perfume ingredients tested using a modified draize procedure. *Toxicology* 9(3):261–271.

1196. Shore RE, Pasternack BS, Thiessen EU, Sadow M, Forbes R, Albert RE. A case-control study of hair dye use and breast cancer. *JNCI* 62(2):277–283, Feb 1979.

1197. Simpson JR. Dermatitis due to parabens in cosmetic creams. *Contact Dermatitis* 4(5):311–312, Oct 1978.

1198. Spencer PS, Sterman AB, Bischoff M, Horoupian D, Foster GV. Experimental myelin disease and ceroid accumulation produced by the fragrance compound acetyl ethyl tetramethyl tetralin. *Tran Am Neurol Assoc* 103:185–187, 1978.

1199. Spencer PS, Sterman AB, Horoupian DS, Foulds MM. Neurotoxic fragrance produces ceroid and myelin disease. *Science* 204(4393):633–635, May 11 1979.

1200. Stavraky KM, Clarke EA, Donner A. Case-control study of hair dye use by patients with breast cancer and endometrial cancer. *J Natl Cancer Inst* 63(4):941–945, Oct 1979.

1201. Suskind RR. Cutaneous reactions to cosmetics. *J Dermatol* (Tokyo) 6(4):203–209, Aug 1979.

1202. Swift DL, Zuskin E, Bouhuys A. Respiratory deposition of hair spray aerosol and acute lung function changes. *Lung* 156(2):149–158, May 18 1979.

1203. Tentative first priority list of cosmetic ingredients for review by the expert panel. *Clin Toxicol* 12(3):381–412, 1978.

1204. Thomas ET, Barton SN. The role of eye cosmetic contaminants in the pathogenesis of eye infection: an epidemilogic investigation. *Ala J Med Sci* 15(3):246–251, Jul 1978.

1205. Tunnessen WW Jr. Perioral dermatitis from a flavored lip balm. *Pediatrics* 63(4):673–674, Apr 1979.

1206. van Abbe NJ. Cosmetic benefit and risk in perspective. *Int J Dermatol* 18(6):461–463, Jul-Aug 1979.

1207. van Ketel WG. Dermatitis from an aftershave. *Contact Dermatitis* 4(2):117, Apr 1978.

1208. van Ketel WG. Patch testing with eye cosmetics. *Contact Dermatitis* 5(6):402, Dec 1979.

1209. Varma BK, Cincotta J. Mouthwash-induced hypoglycemia. *Am J Dis Child* 132(9):930–931, Sep 1978.

1210. Weaver A, Fleming SM, Smith DB. Mouthwash and oral cancer: carcinogen or coincidence? *J Oral Surg* 37(4):250–253, Apr 1979.

1211. Wells IP, Dubbins PA, Whimster WF. Pulmonary disease caused by the inhalation of cosmetic talcum powder. *Br J Radiol* 52(619):586–588, Jul 1979.

Drugs

1212. Alvan G. Individual differences in the disposition of drugs metabolised in the body. *Clin Pharmacokinet* 3(2):155–175, Mar-Apr 1978.

1213. Anderson PO. Drugs and breast feeding. *Semin Perinatol* 3(3):271–278, Jul 1979.

1214. Argov Z, Mastaglia FL. Drug therapy: disorders of neuromuscular transmission caused by drugs. *N Engl J Med* 301(8):409–413, Aug 23 1979. 1979.

1215. Evans L. Psychological effects caused by drugs in overdose. *Drugs* 19(3):220–242, Mar 1980.

1216. Exaire E, Trevino-Becerra A, Monteon F. An overview of treatment with peritoneal dialysis in drug poisoning. *Contrib Nephrol* 17:39–43, 1979.

1217. Fell GS. Toxic metal exposure during medication. *Proc Nutr Soc* 38(2):263–268, Sep 1979.

1218. Filipek WJ. Drug-induced pulmonary disease. *Postgrad Med* 65(2):131–136, 139–140, Feb 1979.

1219. Flaherty JA. Psychiatric complications of medical drugs. *J Fam Pract* 9(2):243–251, Aug 1979.

1220. Green PH, Tall AR. Drugs, alcohol and malabsorption. *Am J Med* 67(6):1066-1076, Dec 1979.

1221. Howard FM, Hill JM. Drugs in pregnancy. *Obstet Gynecol Surv* 34(9):643-653, Sep 1979.

1222. Humphreys DJ. A review of recent trends in animal poisoning. *Br Vet J* 134(2):128-145, Mar-Apr 1978.

1223. Kligman AM. Cutaneous toxicology: an overview from the underside. *Curr Probl Dermatol* 7:1-25, 1978.

1224. Lawson DH. Detection of drug-induced disease. *Br J Clin Pharmacol* 7(1):13-18, Jan 1979.

1225. Levine L. Reported ocular side effects of the ten most frequently prescribed drugs. *J Am Optom Assoc* 50(2):221-227, Feb 1979.

1226. Locket S. Overdose. *Br J Hosp Med* 19(3):200, 205-209, 212, Mar 1978.

1227. Maddrey WC, Boitnott JK. Drug-induced chronic hepatitis and cirrhosis. *Prog Liver Dis* 6:595-603, 1979.

1228. Mettler FA Jr. Manifestations of drug toxicity. *Curr Probl Diagn Radiol* 13(4):1-55, Jul-Aug 1979.

1229. Oehme FW. Poison control in pets. *Vet Hum Toxicol* 21 Suppl:81-88, 1979.

1230. Pond S, Rosenberg J, Benowitz NL, Takki S. Pharmakokinetics of haemoperfusion for drug overdose. *Clin Pharmacokinet* 4(5):329-354, Sep-Oct 1979.

1231. Popper H, Gerber MA, Schaffner F, Selikoff IJ. Environmental hepatic injury in man. *Prog Liver Dis* 6:605-638, 1979.

1232. Salway JG. Drug interference causing misinterpretation of laboratory results. How to solve the problem. *Ann Clin Biochem* 15(1):44-48, Jan 1978,

1233. Smithellis RW. Drugs, infections, and congenital abnormalities. *Arch Dis Child* 53(2):93-99, Feb 1978.

1234. Takki S, Gambertoglio JG, Honda DH, Tozer TN. Pharmacokinetic evaluation of hemodialysis in acute drug overdose. *J Pharmacokinet Biopharm* 6(5):427-442, Oct 1978.

1235. van Berge Hanegouwen GP, Vogten AJ. Drug-induced liver injury. *Neth J Med* 23(1):23-32, 1980.

1236. Wardell WM, Tsianco MC, Anavekar SN, Davis HT. Postmarketing surveillance of new drugs: I. Review of objectives and methodology. *J Clin Pharmacol* 19(2-3):85-94, Feb-Mar 1979.

1237. Wilson FM 2d. Adverse external ocular effects of topical ophthalmic medications. *Surv Ophthalmol* 24(2):57-88, Sep-Oct 1979.

1238. Winchester JF, Gelfand MC, Tilstone WJ. Hemoperfusion in drug intoxication: clinical and laboratory aspects. *Drug Metab Rev* 8(1):69-104, 1978.

1239. Woods HF. Effects of nutrition on drug metabolism and distribution. *Compr Ther* 4(10):49-53, Oct 1978.

Environmental Toxicology

1240. Alford A. Environmental applications of mass spectrometry. *Biomed Mass Spectrum* 5(4):259-286, Apr 1978.

1241. Alvares AP. Research review: interactions between environmental chemicals and drug biotransformation in man. *Clin Pharmacokinet* 3(6):462-477, Nov-Dec 1978.

1242. Anderson HA, Selikoff IJ. Pleural reactions to environmental agents. *Fed Proc* 37(11):2496-2500, Sep 1978.

1243. Aviado DM. Physiological and biochemical responses to specific group of inhalants: concluding remarks. *Fed Proc* 37(11):2508-2509, Sep 1978.

1244. Babich H, Stotzky G. Atmospheric sulfur compounds and microbes. *Environ Res* 15(3):513-531, Jun 1978.

1245. Barnes WS, Klekowski EJ Jr. Testing the environment for dispersed mutagens: use of plant bioconcentrators coupled with microbial mutagen assays. *Environ Health Perspect* 27:61-67, Dec 1978.

1246. Bend JR, James MO, Dansette PM. In vitro metabolism of xenobiotics in some marine animals. *Ann NY Acad Sci* 298:505-521, Sep 29 1978.

1247. Blumberg WE. Enzymic modification of environmental intoxicants: the role of cytochrome P-450. *Q Rev Biophys* 11(4):481-542, Nov 1978.

1248. Bryan GW. Bioaccumulation of marine pollutants. *Phil. Trans R Soc Lond* [*Biol*] 286(1015):483-505, Aug 1979.

1249. Buck WB. Animals as monitors of environmental quality. *Vet Hum Toxicol* 21(4):277-284, Aug 1979.

1250. Cohen HS, Freedman ML, Goldstein BD. The problem of benzene in our environment: clinical and molecular considerations. *Am J Med Sci* 275(2):124-136, Mar-Apr 1978.

1251. Couch JA, Courtney L. Interaction of chemical pollutants and virus in a crustacean: a novel bioassay system. *Ann NY Acad Sci* 298:497-504, Sep 29 1978.

1252. Cucu F. Carbon monoxide and its implications in atherosclerosis etiopathogeny. *Med Interna* 16(3):229-242, Jul-Sep 1978.

1253. Dagley S. Determinants of biodegradability. *Q Rev Biophys* 11(4):577-602, Nov 1978.

1254. Damstra T. Environmental chemicals and nervous system dysfunction. *Yale J Biol Med* 51(4):457–468, Jul-Aug 1978.

1255. Dawson SV, Schenker MB. Health effects of inhalation of ambient concentrations of nitrogen dioxide. *Am Rev Respir Dis* 120(2):281–292, Aug 1979.

1256. Ellison JM, Waller RE. A review of sulphur oxides and particulate matter as air pollutants with particular reference to effects on health in the United Kingdom. *Environ Res* 16(1–3):302–325, Jul 1978.

1257. Ferris BG Jr. Health effects of exposure to low levels of regulated air pollutants: a critical review. *J Air Pollut Control Assoc* 28(5):482–497, May 1978.

1258. Freeling M. Maize Adh1 as a monitor of environmental mutagens. *Environ Health Perspect* 27:91–107, Dec 1978.

1259. Giacoia GP, Catz CS. Drugs and pollutants in breast milk. *Clin Perinatol* 6(1):181–196, Mar 1979.

1260. Grant WF. Chromosome aberrations in plants as a monitoring system. *Environ Health Perspect* 27:37–43, Dec 1978.

1261. Guidotti TL. The higher oxides of nitrogen: inhalation toxicology. *Environ Res* 15(3):443–472, Jun 1978.

1262. Harkonen H. Styrene, its experimental and clinical toxicology: a review. *Scand J Work Environ Health* 4[Suppl 2]:104–113, 1978.

1263. Magos L. Mercury: an environmental and dietary hazard. *J Hum Nutr* 32(3):179–186, Jun 1978.

1264. Malins DC. Metabolism of aromatic hydrocarbons in marine organisms. *Ann NY Acad Sci* 298:482–496, Sep 29 1978.

1265. Mearns AJ, Sherwood MJ. Distribution of neoplasms and other diseases in marine fishes relative to the discharge of waste water. *Ann NY Acad Sci* 298:210–223, Sep 29 1978.

1266. Mercury in the Ottawa River: Ottawa River Project Group. *Environ Res* 19(2):231–243, Aug 1979.

1267. Mulla MS, Majori G, Arata AA. Impact of biological and chemical mosquito control agents on nontarget biota in aquatic ecosystems. *Residue Rev* 71:122–173, 1979.

1268. Nilan RA. Potential of plant genetic systems for monitoring and screening mutagens. *Environ Health Perspect* 27:181–196, Dec 1978.

1269. Nurnberg HW. Polarography and voltammetry in studies of toxic metals in man and his environment. *Sci Total Environ* 12(1):35–60, May 1979.

1270. Odum WE, Drifmeyer JE. Sorption of pollutants by plant detritus: a review. *Environ Health Perspect* 27:133–137, Dec 1978.

1271. Overstreet RM, Howse HD. Some parasites and diseases of estuarine fishes in polluted habitats of Mississippi. *Ann NY Acad Sci* 298:427–462, Sep 29 1978.

1272. Persoone G, Dive D. Toxicity tests on ciliates: a short review. *Ecotoxicol Environ Safety* 2(2):105–114, Sep 1978.

1273. Popper H. Gerber MA, Schaffner F, Selikoff IJ. Environmental hepatic injury in man. *Prog Liver Dis* 6:605–638, 1979.

1274. Robson A. Energy policy and the public health: environmental implications of fossil-fueled power stations. *R Soc Health J* 99(6):247–258, Dec 1979.

1275. Rogan WJ, Bagniewska A, Damstra T. Pollutants in breast milk. *N Engl J Med* 302(26):1450–1453, Jun 1980.

1276. Shephard RJ. Cigarette smoking and reactions to air pollutants. *Can Med Assoc J* 118(4):379–381, 383, 392, Feb 18 1978.

1277. Smith G, Shirley AW. A review of the effects of trace concentrations of anaesthetics on performance. *Br J Anesth* 50(7):701–712, Jul 1978.

1278. Smith WD. Pollution and the anaesthetist. *Int Anesthesiol Clin* 16(1):131–173, Spring 1978.

1279. Trosko JE, Chang C. Genes, pollutants and human diseases. *Q Rev Biophys* 11(4):603–627, Nov 1978.

1280. Van Hook RI. Transport and transportation pathways of hazardous chemicals from solid waste disposal. *Environ Health Perspect* 27:295–308, Dec 1978.

1281. Wassermann M, Wassermann D, Cucos S, Miller HJ. World PCBs map: storage and effects in man and his biologic environment in the 1970s. *Ann NY Acad Sci* 320:69–124, May 31 1979. -PCR's

1282. Weir FW. Toxicology of the sulfur oxides. *JOM* 21(4):281–283, Apr 1979.

1283. Wood RW. Stimulus properties of inhaled substances. *Environ Health Perspect* 26:69–76, Oct 1978.

1284. Zenz C. Benzene: attempts to establish a lower exposure standard in the United States: a review. *Scand J Work Environ Health* 4(2):103–113, Jun 1978.

Food

1285. Arnold SH, Brown WD. Histamine toxicity from fish products. *Adv Food Res* 24:113–154, 1978.

1286. Bahna SL. Control of milk allergy: a challenge for physicians, mothers and industry. *Ann Allergy* 41(1):1–12, Jul 1978.

1287. Bahna SL, Heiner DC. Cow's milk allergy: pathogenesis, manifestations, diagnosis and management. *Adv Pediatr* 25:1-37, 1978.

1288. Barratt ME, Strachan PJ, Porter P. Immunologically mediated nutritional disturbances associated with soya-protein antigens. *Proc Nutr Soc* 38(1):143-150, May 1 1979.

1289. Battarbee HD, Meneely GR. The toxicity of salt. *CRC Crit Rev Toxicol* 5(4):355-376, Sep 1978.

1290. Chan-Yeung M, Ashley MJ, Brzybowski S. Grain dust and the lungs. *Can Med Assoc J* 188(10):1271-1274, May 20 1978.

1291. Constantino D. Mushroom poisoning in Italy. *Int J Artif Organs* 1(6):257-259, Nov 1978.

1292. Cummings JH. Dietary factors in the aetiology of gastrointestinal cancer. *J. Hum Nutr* 32(6):455-465, Dec 1978.

1293. Fries JH. Chocolate: a review of published reports of allergic and other deleterious effects, real or presumed. *Ann Allergy* 41(4):195-207, Oct 1978.

1294. Faulstich H. New aspects of amanita poisoning. *Klin Wochenschr* 57(21):1143-1152, Nov 1979.

1295. Genest J, Nowaczynski W, Boucher R, Kuchel O. Role of the adrenal cortex and sodium in the pathogenesis of human hypertension. *Can Med Assoc J* 188(5):538-549, Mar 4 1978.

1296. Gori GB. Dietary and nutritional implications in the multifactorial etiology of certain prevalent human cancers. *Cancer* 43[Suppl 5]:2151-2161, May 1979.

1297. Gori GB. Role of diet and nutrition in cancer cause, prevention and treatment. *Bull Cancer* (Paris) 65(2):115-126, 1978.

1298. Graham S, Haenszel W, Bock FG, Lyon JL. Need to pursue new leads in the epidemiology of colorectal cancer. *J Natl Cancer Inst* 63(4):879-881, Oct 1979.

1299. Habs M, Schmahl D. Diet and cancer. *J Cancer Res Clin Oncol* 96(1):1-10, Jan 1980.

1300. Khera KS, Munro IC. A review of the specifications and toxicity of synthetic food colors permitted in Canada. *CRC Crit Rev Toxicol* 6(2):81-133, Jan 1979.

1301. Kritchevsky D. Food products and hyperlipidemia. *Arch Surg* 113(1):52-54, Jan 1978.

1302. Lampe KF. Toxic fungi. *Annu Rev Pharmacol Toxicol* 19:85-104, 1979.

1303. Matzkies F, Berg G. Dietary fiber syndrome as the cause of disease in civilized societies. *Acta Hepatogastroenterol* (Stuttg) 25(5):402-407, Oct 1978.

1304. McDonel JL. The molecular mode of action of Clostridium perfringens enterotoxin. *Am J Clin Nutr* 32(1):210–218, Jan 1979.

1305. Newell GR, Hoover RN, Kolbye AC Jr. Status report on saccharin in humans. *JNCI* 61(2):275–276, Aug 1978.

1306. Polin RA, Brown LW. Infant botulism. *Pediatr Clin North Am* 26(2):345–354, May 1979.

1307. Preussmann R. Toxicological aspects of food safety—carcinogenicity and mutagenicity. *Arch Toxicol* (Suppl 1):69–84, 1978.

1308. Ross-Smith P, Jenner FA. Diet (gluten) and schizophrenia. *J Hum Nutr* 34(2):107–112, Apr 1980.

1309. Tobian L. Salt and hypertension. *Ann NY Academ Sci* 304:178–202, Mar 30 1978.

1310. Tobian L. The relationship of salt to hypertension. *Am J Clin Nutr* 32(Suppl 12):2739–2748, Dec 1979.

1311. Turnbull PC. Food poisoning with special reference to Salmonella: its epidemiology, pathogenesis and control. *Clin Gastroenterol* 8(3):663–714, Sep 1979.

1312. Weisburger JH. Mechanism of action of diet as a carcinogen. *Cancer* 43(Suppl 5):1987–1995, May 1979.

1313. Wixom RL, Davis GE, Flynn MA, Tsutakawa RT, Hentges DJ. Excretion of creatine and creatinine in feces of man. *Proc Soc Exp Biol Med* 161(4):452–457, Sep 1979.

Legislative, Regulatory, and Societal Issues

1314. Alston P. International regulation of toxic chemicals. *Ecol Law Quart* 7(2):397–456, 1978.

1315. Baram MS. Radiation from nuclear power plants—need for congressional directives. *Harvard J Legislation* 14(4):905–945, 1977.

1316. Berger JL, Riskin SD. Economic and technological feasibility in regulating toxic substances under the Occupational Safety and Health Act. *Ecol Law Quart* 7(2):285–358, 1978.

1317. Bingham E. Legislative control of toxic hazards. 1. The approach in the USA. *Ann Occup Hyg* 23(1):79–83, 1980.

1318. Biryukova AP. Special protective legislation and equality of opportunity for women workers in the USSR. *Int Labour Rev (Switzerland)* 119(1):51–65, Jan/Feb 1980.

1319. Boyle RH, Highland JH. The persistence of PCBs. *Environment* 21(5):6–13, 37, 1979.

1320. Browning JB. Managing a premanufacture notifcation program. *Hazardous Materials Manag J* 1(4):34–36, May/June 1980.

1321. Calkins DR, Dixon RL, Gerber CR, Zarin D, Omenn GS. Identification, characterization, and control of potential human carcinogens: a framework for Federal decision-making. *JNCI* 64(1):169–176, 1980.

1322. Christensen CN. Federal regulation: philosophy and practice. *Ann Int Med* 89:835–837, Nov (Part 2), 1978.

1323. Cooke MA. Philosophy of cosmetic and toiletry safety evaluation. *Soap Perfum Cosmet* 51:101–102, Mar 1978.

1324. Cordle F, Kolbye AC. Food safety and public health: Interaction of science and law in the Federal regulatory process. *Cancer* 43(5 suppl):2143–2150, 1979.

1325. Croke KG, Raufer RK. Management of toxic chemical spills. *J Air Poll Control Assoc* 28(1):55–57, 1978.

1326. Culliton BJ. Toxic substances legislation: how well are laws being implemented? *Science* 201(4362):1198–1199, 1978.

1327. Desanti RJ. Cost benefit analysis for standards regulating toxic substances under the occupational safety and health act: American Petroleum Institute v. OSHA. *Boston Univ Law R* 60:115–143, Jan 1980.

1328. Dixon RL. United States governmental efforts to improve the regulation of toxic substances. *Arch Toxicol* 43(1):35–45, 1979.

1329. Doniger DD. Federal regulation of vinyl chloride: short course in law and policy of toxic substances control. *Ecol Law Quart* 7(2):497–677, 1978.

1330. Douglas DB. Implications of health and safety legislation. *IARC Sci Publ* 74(25):81–86, 1979.

1331. Draggan S, Giddings JM. Testing toxic substances for protection of the environment. *Sci Total Environ* 9(1):63–74, 1978.

1332. Drobeck HP. Impact of GLP regulations on an industrial toxicology laboratory. *Pharm Tech* 3:35–38, Aug 1979.

1333. Edmunds SW. Economic measures of toxic substance regulation. *Exotoxicol Environ Saf* 3(2):101–110, 1979.

1334. Frankel G. The tragedy of TOSCA: chemical poisoning the EPA can't control. *Washington Mo* 11:42–45, Jul/Aug 1979.

1335. Garrett TL. The law of toxic substances. *Environ Health Perspect* 32:279–284, 1979.

1336. Gaynor K. Toxic Substances Control Act—Regulatory morass. *Vanderbilt Law Rev* 30(6):1149–1195, 1977.

1337. Gelzer J. Governmental toxicology regulations: an encumbrance to drug research? *Arch Toxicol* 43(1):19–26, 1979.

1338. Hall RM. Evolution and implementation of EPA's regulatory program to control discharge of toxic pollutants to nation's waters. *Natural Resources Lawyer* 10(3):507–529, 1977.

1339. Heritage J. Major American toxics disasters. *EPA J* 4(8):8-10, 1978.

1340. Keith LH, Telliard WA. Priority pollutants. 1. A perspective view. *Environ Sci Technol* 13(4):416-443, 1979.

1341. Kappeler TU. The world ecotoxicology watch. *Environ Sci Technol* 13(4):412-415, 1979.

1342. Kmet MA. Movement of hazardous cargo. *Security Mgmt* 24(4):32-34, Apr 1980.

1343. Koch K. Seeping from under the carpet: Cleaning up chemical dumps posing dilemma for congress. *Cong Q W Rept* 38:795-797, Mar 22, 1980.

1344. Kolojeski JC, Murphy MJ. Avoiding toxic chemical liability through preventive analysis. *Risk Mgmt* 27(4):12-16, Apr 1980.

1345. Langley E. Health and safety aspects of the proposed notification scheme for new chemicals. *Chem Ind (London)* 14:504-507, 1978.

1346. Lasagna L. Toxicological barriers to providing better drugs. *Arch Toxicol* 43(1):27-33, 1979.

1347. Latarjet R. Regulation of radiation pollution: Its possible usefulness in strategy for intervention against chemical mutagens. *IARC Sci Publ* 25:207-228, 1979.

1348. Leepson, M. Toxic substance control. *Editorial Res. Rep* 743-760, Oct 13 1978.

1349. Leimgruber R. International legislation regarding toxics. *Chimia* 32(10):403-405, 1978.

1350. Lepore PD. FDA's Good Laboratory Practice regulations. *Pharm Tech* 3:71-74, June 1979.

1351. Linsell CA. Decision on the control of a dietary carcinogen—aflatoxin. *IARC Sci Publ* 74(25):111-122, 1979.

1352. Massey KA. Challenge of nonionizing radiation: proposal for legislation. *Duke Law J* 1979(1):105-189, 1979.

1353. Maxey MN. Radiation protection philosophy: bioethical problems and priorities. *Am Ind Hyg Assoc J* 39(9):689-694, 1978.

1354. McGarity TO. Substantive and procedural discretion in administrative resolution of science policy questions—regulating carcinogens in EPA and OSHA. *Georgetown Law J* 67(3):729-810, 1979.

1355. McLean AE. Hazards from chemicals: scientific questions and conflicts of interest. *Proc R Soc Lond (Biol)* 205(1158):179-197, 1979.

1356. McNamara BP. Concepts and methodology for toxicological testing. *ACS Symp Ser* 96:215-236, 1979.

1357. Merrill RA. Regulating carcinogens in food: legislators guide to the food safety provisions of the Federal Food, Drug, and Cosmetic Act. *Michigan Law Review* 77(2):171–250, 1978.

1358. Nemec MM. Amend OSHA forces will gain momentum in 1980. *Occupational Hazards* 41(12):41–44, Dec 1979.

1359. Page T. Generic view of toxic chemicals and similar risks. *Ecology Law Quarterly* 7(2):207–244, 1978.

1360. Perkins JL, Rose VE. Occupational health priorities for health standards: the current NIOSH approach. *Am J Public Health* 69(5):444–448, 1979.

1361. Pittom LA. Legislative control of toxic hazards. 2. The approach in the UK. *Annals of Occupational Hygiene* 23(1):85–90, 1980.

1362. Proposed system for food safety assessment. Scientific Committee, Food Safety Council. *Food Cosmet Toxicol* 16(2):1–136, 1978.

1363. Risk benefit analysis and technology-forcing under Toxic Substances Control Act. *Iowa Law Rev* 62(3):942–959, 1977.

1364. Robens JF. Criteria for deciding the need for chronic testing: a regulatory viewpoint. *Vet Hum Toxicol* 21(6):427–430, 1979.

1365. Ruttenberg R. As the economy changes—so must our economic decision making. *Hazardous Materials Manag J* 1(4):11–19, May/June 1980.

1366. Shapiro SA. The trade secret status of health and safety testing information: reforming agency disclosure policies. *Harvard Law R* 93:837–888, Mar 1980.

1367. Sittig M. Legislation bearing on toxic hazards of industrial chemicals. *Occup Health Saf* 48(7):64–65, 1979.

1368. Smith RJ. Toxic substances: EPA and OSHA are reluctant regulators. *Science* 203(4375):28–32, 1979.

1369. Soble SM. A proposal for the administrative compensation of victims of toxic substance pollution: A model act. *Harvard J Legislation* 14:683–824, Jun 1977.

1370. Somers E. Risk assessment for environmental health. *Can J Public Health* 70(6):388–392, 1979.

1371. Sprout WL. How do you inform labor, management, and other professionals about toxicity data? *Occup Health Saf* 47(2):20–21, 1978.

1372. Symposium on ''Impact of Toxicological Regulations on Modern Society,'' 26 May 1978, Rome. *Arch Toxicol* 43(1):1–45, 1979.

1373. Tiefer C. OSHA's toxics program faces a Supreme Court test. *Labor Law J* 30:680–688, Nov 1979.

1374. Wallis RR, Hartfield JA, Wiersema J. The regulation of toxic air pollutants in Texas. *Tex Rep Biol Med* 37:191–203, 1978.

1375. Walsh J. EPA and toxic substances law: dealing with uncertainty. *Science* 202 (4368):602–604, 1978.

1376. Weinberg AM. The nuclear management syndrome. *Wharton Mag* 4(1):20–27, Fall 1979.

1377. Winkler NT. Administering and enforcing radiation control. *Radiol Technol* 50(6):731–733, May-Jun 1979.

1378. Witt M. Dangerous substances and the US worker: current practice and viewpoints. *Int Labour R* 118(2):165–177, Mar-Apr 1979.

1379. Woods JS. Epidemiologic considerations in the design of toxicologic studies—approach to risk assessment in humans. *Fed Proc* 38(5):1891–1896, 1979.

1380. Wynder EL. Cultural and behavioral aspects of risk-factors: society's obligation. *J Environ Pathol Toxicol* 1(2):11–18, 1977.

1381. Young ML. Legal responsibility of the scientist in handling data. *Clin Toxicol* 15(5):605–611, 1979.

1382. Zener RV. Toxic Substances Control Act: Federal regulation of commercial chemicals. *Bus Lawyer* 32(4):1685–1703, 1977.

Metals

1383. Alvares AP, Kappas A. Lead and polychlorinated biphenyls: effects on heme and drug metabolism. *Drug Metab Rev* 10(1):91–106 1979.

1384. Babich H, Stotzky G. Effects of cadmium on the biota: influence of environmental factors. *Adv Appl Microbiol* 23:55–117, 1978.

1385. Ban TA. Adverse effects in maintenance therapy. *Int Pharmacopsychiatry* 13(4):217–29, 1978.

1386. Battarbee HD, Meneely GR. The toxicity of salt. *CRC Crit Rev Toxicol.* 5(4):355–76, Sep 1978.

1387. Bergman JJ, Rosen GD, Moeller DA. Appendicitis associated with recent barium study. *J Fam Pract* 8(5):931–935, May 1979.

1388. Bremner I. The toxicity of cadmium, zinc and molybdenum and their effects on copper metabolism. *Proc Nutr Soc* 38(2):235–242, Sep 1979.

1389. Constantinidis K. Acute and chronic beryllium disease. *Br J Clin Pract* 32(5):127–136, 153, May 1978.

1390. Factors influencing metabolism and toxicity of metals: a consensus report. *Environ Health Perspect* 25:3–41, Aug 1978.

1391. Fell GS. Toxic metal exposure during medication. *Proc Nutr Soc* 38(20):263–268, Sep 1979.

1392. Genest J, Nowaczynski W, Boucher R, Kuchel O. Role of the adrenal cortex and sodium in the pathogenesis of human hypertension. *Can Med Assoc J* 118(5):538–549, Mar 4 1978.

1393. Gibbons RB. Complications of chrysotherapy: a review of recent studies. *Arch Intern Med* 139(3):343–346, Mar 1979.

1394. Grandjean P, Nielson T. Organolead compounds: environmental health aspects. *Residue Rev* 72:97–148, 1979.

1395. Granoff AL, Davis JM. Heal illness syndrome and lithium intoxication. *J Clin Psychiatr* 39(2):103–107, Feb 1978.

1396. Hansen HE, Amdisen A. Lithium intoxication: report of 23 cases and review of 100 cases from the literature. *Q J Med* 47(186):123–144, Apr 1978.

1397. Harrist TJ, Schiller AL, Trelstad RL, Mankin HJ, Mays CW. Thorotrast-associated sarcoma: a case report and review of the literature. *Cancer* 44(6):2049–2058, Dec 1979.

1398. Havdala HS, Borison RL, Diamond BI. Potential hazards and applications of lithium in anesthesiology. *Anesthesiology* 50(6):534–537, Jun 1979.

1399. Hwang S, Tuason VB. Long-term maintenance lithium therapy and possible irreversible renal damage. *J Clin Psych.* 41(1):11–19, Jan 1980.

1400. Jones PA, Taintor JF, Adams AB. Comparative dental material cytotoxicity measured by depression of rat incisor pulp respiration. *J Endod* 5(2):48–55, Feb 1979.

1401. Krigman MR. Neuropathology of heavy metal intoxication. *Environ Health Perspect* 26:117–120, Oct 1978.

1402. Madias NE, Harrington JT. Platinum nephrotoxicity. *Am J Med* 65(2):307–314, Aug 1978.

1403. Maines MD. Role of trace metals in regulation of cellular heme and hemoprotein metabolism: sensitizing effects of chronic iron treatment on acute gold toxicity. *Drug Metab Rev* 9(2):237–255, 1979.

1404. McNerney RT, McNerney JJ. Mercury contamination in the dental office. *NY State Dent J* 45(9):457–458, Nov 1979.

1405. Modell B. Advances in the use of iron-chelating agents for the treatment of iron overload. *Prog Hematol* 11:267–312, 1979.

1406. Payne BJ, Saunders LZ. Heavy metal nephropathy of rodents. *Vet Pathol* 15[Suppl 5]:51–87, Aug 1978.

1407. Shabalina LP, Spiridonova VS. Thallium as an industrial poison: review of literature. *J Hyg Epidemiol Microbiol Immunol* (Praha) 23(3):247–255, 1979.

1408. Shannon IL. Stannous flouride: does it stain teeth? How does it react with tooth surfaces? A review. *Gen Dent* 26(5):64–71, Sept-Oct 1978.

1409. Sindelar WF, Costa J, Ketcham AS. Osteosarcoma associated with Thorotrast administration: report of two cases and literature review. *Cancer* 42(6):2604–2609, Dec 1978.

1410. Soli NE. Chronic copper poisoning in sheep. A review of the literature. *Nord Vet Med* 32(2):75–89, Feb 1980.

1411. Sunderman FW Jr. Carcinogenic effects of metals. *Fed Proc* 37(1):40–46 Jan 1978.

1412. Taylor D. A review of the lethal and sub-lethal effects of mercury on aquatic life. *Residue Rev* 72:33–69, 1979.

1413. Tephly TR, Wagner G, Sedman R, Piper W. Effects of metals on heme biosynthesis and metabolism. *Fed Proc* 37(1):35–39, Jan 1978.

1414. Thomsen K. Olesen OV. Precipitating factors and renal mechanisms in lithium intoxication. *Gen Pharmacol* 9(2):85–89, 1978.

1415. Tobian L. Salt and hypertension. *Ann NY Acad Sci* 304:178–202, Mar 30 1978.

1416. Tobian L. The relationship of salt to hypertension. *Am J Clin Nutr* 32[Suppl 12]:2739–2748, Dec 1979.

1417. Von Hoff DD, Schilsky R, Reichert CM, Reddick RL, Rozencweig M, Young RC, Muggia FM. Toxic effects of cis-dichlorodiammine-platinum (II) in man. *Cancer Treat Rep* 63(9-10):1527–1531, Sep-Oct 1979.

1418. Waldron HA. Lead and human behavior. *J Ment Defic Res* 22(1):69–78, Mar 1978.

1419. Ward GM. Molybdenum toxicity and hypocuprosis in ruminants: a review. *J Anim Sci* 46(4):1078–1085, Apr 1978.

1420. Weiss B. The behavioral toxicology of metals. *Fed Proc* 37(1):22–27, Jan 1978.

Occupational Health and Industrial Hygiene

1421. Abraham JL. Recent advances in pneumonconiosis: the pathologist's role in etiologic diagnosis. *Monogr Pathol* 19:96–137, 1978.

1422. Aschoff J. Features of circadian rhythms relevant for the design of shift schedules. *Ergonomics* 21(10):739–754, Oct 1978.

1423. Back KC, Carter VL Jr. Thomas AA. Occupational hazards of missile operations with special regard to the hydrazine propellants. *Aviat Space Environ Med* 49(4):592–598, Apr 1978.

1424. Binns CH. Vinyl chloride: a review. *J Soc Occup Med* 29(4):134–141, Oct 1979.

1425. Chan-Yeung M, Ashley MJ. Grzybowski S. Grain dust and the lungs. *Can Med Assoc J* 118(10):1271–1274, May 20 1978.

1426. Chovil AC. Occupational lung cancer and smoking: a review in the light of current theories of carcinogenesis. *Can Med Assoc J* 121(5):548-550, 553-555, Sep 8 1979.

1427. Constantinidis K. Acute and chronic beryllium disease. *Br J Clin Pract* 32(5):127-136, 153, May 1978.

1428. Feldman NT, McFadden ER Jr. Occupational asthma. *Compr Ther* 4(4):23-28, Apr 1978.

1429. Freundt KJ. Nervous system responses to work-site chemicals: toxicological basis. *Toxicol Eur Res* 1(3):133-144, May 1978.

1430. Guidotti TL. Coal workers' penumoconiosis and medical aspects of coal mining. *South Med J* 72(4):456-466, Apr 1979.

1431. Guidotti TL. The higher oxides of nitrogen: inhalation toxicology. *Environ Res* 15(3):443-472, Jun 1978.

1432. Hemminki K. Sorsa M, Vainio H. Genetic risks caused by occupational chemicals: use of experimental methods and occupational risk group monitoring in the detection of environmental chemicals causing mutations, cancer and malformations. *Scand J Work Environ Health* 5(4):307-327, Dec 1979.

1433. Heppleston AG. Silica and asbestos: contrasts in tissue response. *Ann NY Acad Sci* 330:725-755, 1979.

1434. Kurppa K, Waris P, Rokkanen P. Peritendinitis and tenosynovitis: a review. *Scand J Work Environ Health* 5(3):19-24, 1979.

1435. Levine RJ. How the industrial physician can reduce mortality from asbestos-related diseases. *JOM* 20(7):464-468, Jul 1978.

1436. Liddell FD, Morgan WK. Methods of assessing serial films of the pneumoconioses: a review. *J Soc Occup Med* 28(1):6-15, Jan 1978.

1437. Lutsky I, Toshner D. A review of allergic respiratory disease in laboratory animal workers. *Lab Anim Sci* 28(6):751-756, Dec 1978.

1438. Morgan WK. Industrial bronchitis. *Br J Ind Med* 35(4):285-291, Nov 1978.

1439. Pathology standards for coal workers' pneumoconiosis: report of the Pneumoconiosis Committee of the College of American Pathologists to the National Institute for Occupational Safety and Health. *Arch Pathol Lab Med* 103(8):375-432, Jul 6, 1979.

1440. Pike RM. Laboratory-associated infections: incidence, fatalities, causes, and prevention. *Ann Rev Microbiol* 33:41-66, 1979.

1441. Raven PB, Dodson A, Davis TO. Stresses involved in wearing PVC supplied air suits: a review. *Am Ind Hyg Assoc J* 40(7):592-599, Jul 1979.

1442. Reiser KM, Last JA. Silicosis and fibrogenesis: fact and artifact. *Toxicology* 13(1):51–72, May 1979.

1443. Salvaggio JE. Immunological mechanisms in pulmonary diseases. *Clin Allergy* 9(6):659–668, Nov 1979.

1444. Shabalina LP, Spiridonova VS. Thallium as an industrial poison: review of the literature. *J Hyg Epidemiol Microbiol Immunol* (Praha) 23(3):247–255, 1979.

1445. Schenker MB. Diesel exhaust: an occupational carcinogen? *JOM* 22(1):41–46, Jan 1980.

1446. Smith WD. Pollution and the anaesthetist. *Int Anesthesiol Clin* 16(1):131–173, Spring 1978.

1447. Spence AA, Knill-Jones RP. Is there a health hazard in anaesthetic practice? *Br J Anaesth* 50(7):713–719, Jul 1978.

1448. Tell RA, Harlen F. A review of selected biological effects and dosimetric data useful for development of radiofrequency safety standards for human exposure. *J Microwave Power* 14(4):405–424, Dec 1979.

1449. Tomatis L, Agthe C, Bartsch H, Huff J, Montesano R, Saracci R, Walker E, Wilbourn J. Evaluation of the carcinogenicity of chemicals: a review of the Monograph Program of the International Agency for Research on Cancer (1971 to 1977). *Cancer Res* 38(4):877–885.

1450. Vessey MP. Epidemiological studies of the occupational hazards of anaesthesia: a review. *Anaesthesia* 33(5):430–438, May 1978.

1451. Waldron HA. Target organs: the blood. *J Soc Occup Med* 29(2):65–71, Apr 1979.

1452. Waris P. Occupational cervicobrachial syndromes: a review. *Scand J Work Environ Health* 5(3):3–14, 1979.

1453. Waris P, Kuorinka I, Kurppa K, Luopajarvi T, Virolainen M, Pesonen K, Nummi J, Jukkonen R. Epidemiologic screening of occupational neck and upper limb disorders: methods and criteria. *Scand J Work Environ Health* 5(3):25–38, 1979.

1454. Weisburger JH. Environmental cancer: on the causes of the main human cancers. *Tex Rep Biol Med* 37:1–20, 1978.

1455. Wickstrom G. Effect of work on degenerative back disease: a review. *Scand J Work Environ Health* 4[Suppl 1]:1–12, 1978.

1456. Withers JA. Hepatitis. A review of the disease and its significance to dentistry. *J Periodontol* 51(3):162–166, Mar 1980.

1457. Young RJ, McKay WJ, Evans JM. Coal gasification and occupational health. *Am Ind Hyg Assoc J* 39(12):985–997, Dec 1978.

1458. Zenz C. The epidemiology of carbon monoxide in cardiovascular disease in industrial environments: a review. *Prev Med* 8(3):279–288, May 1979.

Pesticides

1459. Adam SE. Toxicity of indigenous plants and agricultural chemicals in farm animals. *Clin Toxicol* 13(2):269–280, 1978.

1460. Byard JL. Mechanisms of acute human poisoning by pesticides. *Clin Toxicol* 14(2):187–193, 1979.

1461. Chambers J. An introduction to the metabolism of pyrethroids. *Residue Res* 73:101–124, 1980.

1462. Chlordane. *IARC Monogr Eval Carcinog Risk Chem Hum* 20:45–65, Oct 1979.

1463. Dasta JF. Paraquat poisoning: a review. *Am J Hosp Pharm* 35(11):1368–1372, Nov 1978.

1464. Davies JE. Agromedical approach to pesticide management. *Annu Rev Entomol* 23:353–387, 1978.

1465. Dichlorvos. *IARC Monogr Eval Carcinog Risk Chem Hum* 20:97–127, Oct 1979.

1466. Doherty JD. Insecticides affecting ion transport. *Pharmacol Ther* 7(1):123–151, 1979.

1467. Dorough HW. Metabolism of insecticides by conjugation mechanisms. *Pharmacol Ther* 4(2):433–471, 1979.

1468. Egekeze JO, Oehme FW. Sodium monofluoroacetate (SMFA, compound 1080): a literature review. *Vet Hum Toxicol* 21(6):411–416, Dec 1979.

1469. Engst R, Macholz RM, Kujawa M. Recent state of lindane metabolism. Part II. *Residue Rev* 72:71–95, 1979.

1470. Epstein SS. Kepone: hazard evaluation. *Sci Total Environ* 9(1):1–62, Jan 1978.

1471. Fishbein L. Overview of potential mutagenic problems posed by some pesticides and their trace impurities. *Environ Health Perspect* 27:125–131, Dec 1978.

1472. Gupta PK, Gupta RC. Pharmacology, toxicology and degradation of endosulfan: a review. *Toxicology* 13(2):115–130, Jun-Jul 1979.

1473. Haley TJ. A review of the literature of rotenone. *J Environ Pathol Toxicol* 1(3):315–337, Jan-Feb 1978.

1474. Haley TJ. Review of the toxicology of paraquat. *Clin Toxicol* 14(1):1–46, 1979.

1475. Heptachlor and heptachlor epoxide. *IARC Monogr Eval Carcinog Risk Chem Hum* 20:129–154, Oct 1979.

1476. Hexachlorobenzene. *IARC Monogr Eval Carcinog Risk Chem Hum* 20:155–178, Oct 1979.

1477. Hexachlorocyclohexane (technical HCH and lindane). *IARC Monogr Eval Carcinog Risk Chem Hum* 20:195–239, Oct 1979.

1478. Holmstedt B, Nordgren I, Sandoz M, Sundwall A. Metrifonate: summary of toxicological and pharmacological information available. *Arch Toxicol* 41(1):3–29, Oct 13 1978.

1479. Huff JE, Gerstner HB. Kepone: a literature summary. *J Environ Pathol Toxicol* 1(4):377–395, Mar-Apr 1978.

1480. Kapadia SB, Krause JR. Ovarian carcinoma terminating in acute nonlymphocytic leukemia following alkylating agent therapy. *Cancer* 41(5):1676–1679, May 1978.

1481. Labrecque GC, Fye RL. Cytogenetic and other effects of the chemosterilants tepa, metepa, apholate and hempa in insects: a review. *Mutat Res* 47(2):99–113, 1978.

1482. Lal R, Saxena DM. Cytological and biochemical effects of pesticides on microorganisms. *Residue Rev* 73:49–86, 1980.

1483. Manzo L, Gregotti C, Di Nucci A, Richelmi P. Toxicology of paraquat and related bipyridyls: biochemical, clinical and therapeutic aspects. *Vet Hum Toxicol* 21(6):404–410, Dec 1979.

1484. Matthews HB. Excretion of insecticides. *Pharmacol Ther [B]* 4(3): 657–675, 1979.

1485. Menn JJ. Comparative aspects of pesticide metabolism in plants and animals. *Environ Health Perspect* 27:113–124, Dec 1978.

1486. Methoxychlor. *IARC Monogr Eval Carcinog Risk Chem Hum* 20:259–281, Oct 1979.

1487. Mirex. *IARC Monogr Eval Carcinog Risk Chem Hum* 20:283–301, Oct 1979.

1488. Mulla MS, Majori G, Arata AA. Impact of biological and chemical mosquito control agents on nontarget biota in aquatic ecosystems. *Residue Rev* 71:122–173, 1979.

1489. Munnecke DM. Chemical, physical, and biological methods for the disposal and detoxifaction of pesticides. *Residue Rev* 70:1–26, 1979.

1490. Olander K, Haik KG, Haik GM. Management of pterygia: should thiotepa be used? *Ann Ophthalmol* 10(7):853–862, Jul 1978.

1491. Pentachlorophenol. *IARC Monogr Eval Carcinog Risk Chem Hum* 20:303–325, Oct 1979.

1492. Pollock GA, Kilgore WW. Toxaphene. *Residue Rev* 69:87–140, 1978.

1493. Reuber MD. Carcinogenicity of endrin. *Sci Total Environ* 72(2):101–35, Jun 1979.

1494. Reuber MD. Carcinogenicity of kepone. *J Toxicol Environ Health* 4(5-6):895–911, Sep-Nov 1978.

1495. Reuber MD. The carcinogenicity of kepone. *J Environ Pathol Toxicol* 2(3):671–686, Jan-Feb 1979.

1496. Reuber MD. Carcinogenicity of lindane. *Environ Res* 19(2):460–481, Aug 1979.

1497. Reuber MD. Carcinogenicity of toxaphene: a review. *J Toxicol Environ Health* 5(4):729–748, Jul 1979.

1498. Rogan WJ, Bagniewska A, Damstra T. Pollutants in breast milk. *N Engl J Med* 302(26):1450–1453, Jun 1980.

1499. Seiler JP. The genetic toxicology of phenoxy acids other than 2,4,5-T. *Mutat Res* 55(3-4):197–226, 1978.

1500. Sternberg SS. The carcinogenesis, mutagenesis and teratogenesis of insecticides: review of studies in animals and man. *Pharmacol Ther* 6(1):147–166, 1979.

1501. Sub-threshold levels of dietary chemicals and mixed function oxidase induction. *Nutr Rev* 36(4):116–118, Apr 1978.

1502. Thornburg W. Pesticide residues. *Anal Chem* 51(5):196R–210R, Arp 1979.

1503. Toxaphene (polychlorinated camphenes). *IARC Monogr Eval Carcinog Risk Chem Hum* 20:327–348, Oct 1979.

1504. Swietlinska Z, Zuk J. Cytotoxic effects of maleic hydrazide. *Mutat Res* 55(1):15–30, 1978.

1505. Tucker RK, Leitzke JS. Comparative toxicology of insecticides for vertebrate wildlife and fish. *Pharmacol Ther* 6(1):167–220, 1979.

1506. Varela G, Andujar MM, Navarro MP. Chlorinated hydrocarbon insecticides and nutrition. *Worl Rev Nutr Diet* 30:148–188, 1978.

1507. Wassermann M, Wassermann D, Cucos S, Miller HJ. World PCBs map: storage and effects in man and his biologic environment in the 1970s. *Ann NY Acad Sci* 320:69–124, May 31 1979.

1508. Wouters W, van den Bercken J. Action of pyrethroids. *Gen Pharmacol* 9(6):387–398, 1978.

1509. Wright AS, Hutson DH, Wooder MF. The chemical and biochemical reactivity of dichlorvos. *Arch Toxicol* 42(1):1–18, Apr 23 1979.

1510. Zacharski LR, Henderson WG, Rickles FR, Forman WB, Cornell CJ Jr, Forcier RJ, Harrower HW, Johnson RO. Rationale and experimental design for the VA Cooperative Study of Anticoagulation (Warfarin) in the Treatment of Cancer. *Cancer* 44(2):732–741, Aug 1979.

Radiation

1511. Adams GE, Jameson DG. Time effects in molecular radiation biology. *Radiat Environ Biphys* 17(2):95–113, Feb 1980.

1512. Aristizabal SA, Boone ML, Laguna JF. Endocrine factors influencing radiation injury to central nervous tissue. *Int J Radiat Oncol Biol Phys* 5(3):349–353, Mar 1979.

1513. Auclerc G, Jacquillat C, Auclerc MF, Weil M, Bernard J. Post-therapeutic acute leukemia. *Cancer* 44(6):2017–2025, Dec 1979.

1514. Bengtsson G. Maxillo-facial aspects of radiation protection, focused on recent research regarding critical organs. *Dentomaxillofac Radiol* 7(1):5–14, 1978.

1515. Bisby RH, Cundall RB, Davies AK. Aspects of chemical damage in radiation and photo-biology. *Photochem Photobiol* 28(4–5):825–837, Oct-Nov 1978.

1516. Brady LW. Radiation-induced sarcomas of bone. *Skeletal Radiol* 4(2):72–78, Jun 1979.

1517. Burger PC, Mahley MS Jr, Dudka L, Vogel FS. The morphologic effects of a radiation administered therapeutically for intracranial gliomas: a postmortem study of 25 cases. *Cancer* 44(4):1256–1272, Oct 1979.

1518. Carpenter JS. Dental care for children who have received head and neck therapeutic radiation. *J Pedod* 3(1):36–51, Fall 1978.

1519. Catane R, Schwade JG, Turrisi AT 3d, Webber BL, Muggia FM. Pulmonary toxicity after radiation and bleomycin: a review. *Int J Radiat Oncol Biol Phys* 5(9):1513–1518, Sep 1979.

1520. Chen KT, Hoffman, KD, Hendricks EJ. Angiosarcoma following therapeutic irradiation. *Cancer* 44(6):2044–2048, Dec 1979.

1521. D'Angio GJ. Complications of treatment encountered in lymphoma-leukemia long-term survivors. *Cancer* 42(2 Suppl):1015–1025, Aug 1978.

1522. Donaldson SS, Lenon RA. Alterations of nutritional status: impact of chemotherapy and radiation therapy. *Cancer* 43(5 Suppl):2036–2052, May 1979.

1523. Epstein JH. Photocarcinogenesis: a review. *Natl Cancer Inst Monogr* 50:13–25, Dec 1978.

1524. Ergun H, Howland WJ. Postradiation atrophy of mature bone. *CRC Crit Rev Diagn Imaging* 12(3):225–243, Jan 1980.

1525. Evans MJ, Hughes SP. Post-irradiation sarcoma of the clavicle: a report of two patients. *Clin Oncol* 4(2):131–138, Jun 1978.

1526. Fajardo LF, Berthrong M. Radiation injury in surgical pathology. Part I. *Am J Surg Pathol* 2(2):159–199, Jun 1978.

1527. Field SB, Michalowski A. Endpoints for damage to normal tissues. *Int J Radiat Oncol Biol Phys* 5(8):1185–1196, Aug 1979.

1528. Getaz EP, Shimaoka K, Rao U. Anaplastic carcinoma of the thyroid following external irradiation. *Cancer* 43(6):2248–2253, Jun 1979.

1529. Getaz EP, Shimaoka K. Anaplastic carcinoma of the thyroid in a population irradiated for Hodgkin Disease, 1910-1960. *J Surg Oncol* 12(2):181-189, 1979.

1530. Glaeser RM, Taylor KA. Radiation damage relative to transmission electron microscopy of biological specimens at low temperature: a review. *J Microsc* 112(1):127-138, Jan 1978.

1531. Green AE, Hedinger RA. Models relating ultraviolet light and nonmelanoma skin cancer incidence. *Photochem Photobio* 28(2):283-291, Aug 1978.

1532. Griffith RV, Hankins DE, Gammage RB, Tommasino L, Wheeler RV. Recent developments in personnel neutron dosimeters: a review. *Health Phys* 36(3):235-260, Mar 1979.

1533. Haran-Ghera N, Peled A. Induction of leukemia in mice by irradiation and radiation leukemia virus variants. *Adv Cancer Res* 30:45-87, 1979.

1534. Harrist ·TJ, Schiller AL, Trelstad RL, Mankin HJ, Mays CW. Thorotrast-associated sarcoma of bone: a case report and review of the literature. *Cancer* 44(6):2049-2058, Dec 1979.

1535. Hazel JJ. Radiation and the induction of malignancy. *Clin Nucl Med* 4(2):84-85, Feb 1979.

1536. Howell DA. Radiation myelopathy. *Dev Med Child Neurol* 21(5):653-656, Oct 1979.

1537. Kaplan HS. Historic milestones in radiobiology and radiation therapy. *Semin Oncol* 6(4):479-489, Dec 1979.

1538. Koranda JJ, Robison WL. Accumulation of radionuclides by plants as a monitor system. *Environ Health Perspect* 27:165-179, Dec 1978.

1539. Koteles GJ. New aspects of cell membrane radiobiology and their impact on radiation protection *At Energy Rev* 17(1):3-30, Mar 1979.

1540. Kripke ML. Speculations on the role of ultraviolet radiation in the development of malignant melanoma. *JNCI* 63(3):541-548, Sep 1979.

1541. Kwon TH, Boronow RC. Urinary undiversion: use in management of radiation induced bladder fistula. *Gynecol Oncol* 8(2):164-171, Oct 1979.

1542. Localio SA, Pachter HL, Gouge TH. The radiation-injured bowel. *Surg Annu* 11:181-205, 1979.

1543. Manz HJ, Woolley PV 3d, Ornitz RD. Delayed radiation necrosis of brainstem related to fast neutron beam irradiation: case report and literature review. *Cancer* 44(2):473-479, Aug 1979.

1544. Markoe AM. The effects of combined radiation therapy and chemotherapy on the immune response. *Prog Exp Tumor Res* 25:219-228, 1980.

1545. Miller RW. Environmental causes of cancer in childhood. *Adv Pediatr* 25:97-119, 1978.

1546. Mole RH. The sensitivity of the human breast to cancer induction by ionizing radiation. *Br J Radiol* 51(606):401-415, Jun 1978.

1547. Pizzo PA, Poplack DG, Bleyer WA. Neurotoxicities of current leukemia therapy. *Am J Pediatr Hematol Oncol* 1(2):127-140, Summer 1979.

1548. Shaw MT, Spector MH, Ladman AJ. Effects of cancer, radiotherapy and cytotoxic drugs on intestinal structure and function. *Cancer Treat Rev* 6(3):141-151, Sep 1979.

1549. Sindelar WF, Costa J, Ketcham AS. Osteosarcoma associated with thorotrast administration: report of two cases and literature review. *Cancer* 42(6):2604-2609, Dec 1978.

1550. Stenback WA, Bryan ME, Trentin JJ. Radiation carcinogenesis in the Syrian hamster. *Prog Exp Tumor Res* 23:89-99, 1979.

1551. Stewart AM. Cancer effects of low-level radiation: theoretic considerations in competing causes of death. *NY State J Med* 80(1):32-35, Jan 1980.

1552. Stockwell RM. Irradiation related thyroid cancer. History and current recommendations. *Conn Med* 43(2):63-67, Feb 1979.

1553. Tell RA. Harlen, F. A review of selected biological effects and dosimetric data useful for development of radiofrequency safety standards for human exposure. *J Microwave Power* 14(4):405-424, Dec 1979.

1554. Tountas AA, Fornasier VL, Harwood AR, Leung PM. Postirradiation sarcoma of bone: a perspective. *Cancer* 43(1):182-187, Jan 1979.

1555. Turesson I, Notter G. The response of pig skin to single and fractionated high dose-rate and continuous low dose-rate 137Cs-irradiation. II. Theoretical considerations of the results. *Int J Radiat Oncol Biol Phys* 5(7):955-963, Jul 1979.

1556. White DR. Tissue substitutes in experimental radiation physics. *Med Phys* 5(6):467-479, Nov-Dec 1978.

1557. Witt TR, Meng RL, Economou SG, Southwick HW. The approach to the irradiated thyroid. *Surg Clin North Am* 59(1):45-63, Feb 1979.

Appendix I

Directory of Poison Control Centers

This directory has been compiled by the National Clearinghouse for Poison Control Centers and is based on information obtained from the Centers and State Departments of Health. The list also appears in the *Bulletin— National Clearinghouse for Poison Control Centers* 24(8), Aug 1980.

ALABAMA

STATE COORDINATOR
205 832-3194

Department of Public Health
Montgomery 36117

ANNISTON
N.E. Alabama Regional
Medical Center
400 E. 10th St. 36201
205 237-5421   Ext. 307

AUBURN
Auburn University
School of Pharmacy
36830
205 826-4037

BIRMINGHAM
Children's Hospital
1601 6th Ave., S. 35233
205 933-4000

DOTHAN
Southeast Alabama
Medical Center
36301
205 794-3131

FLORENCE
Eliza Coffee
Memorial Hospital
P.O. Box 1079
35630
205 767-1111   Ext. 2045, 2046

GADSDEN
Baptist Memorial Hosp.
1007 Goodyear Avenue
35903
205 492-8111

HUNTSVILLE
    Huntsville Hospital
    101 Sivley Road
    35801
205 539-6320

MOBILE
    University of So. Alabama
        Medical Center
    2451 Fillingim St., 36617
205 473-3325

OPELIKA
    Lee County Hospital
    2000 Pepperill Parkway
    36801
205 749-3411   Ext. 258

TUSKEGEE
    John A. Andrews Hosp.
    Tuskegee Institute
    36088
205 727-8583

ALASKA

STATE   Department of Health & Social Services
COORDINATOR   Juneau 99811
907 465-3100

ANCHORAGE
    Anchorage Poison Center
    Providence Hospital
    3200 Providence Dr.
    99504
907 274-6535

ARIZONA

STATE   Arizona Poison Control System
COORDINATOR   College of Pharmacy
602 626-6016   Tucson 85724

FLAGSTAFF
    Flagstaff Hospital and Med.
        Ctr. of Northern Arizona
    1215 N. Beaver St.
    86001
602 774-5233

TUCSON
    Arizona Poison & Drug
        Information Center
    Arizona Hlth. Sciences Ctr.
    University of Arizona
    85724
    602 626-6016
    1-800 362-0101   (In Arizona)

PHOENIX
    St. Luke's Hospital and
        Medical Center
    525 N. 18th St. 85006
602 253-3334

YUMA
    Yuma Regional Medical Center
    Avenue A and 24 Street
    85364
602 344-2000

230

ARKANSAS

STATE
COORDINATOR
501 661-2397

Department of Health
Little Rock 72201

EL DORADO
Warner Brown Hospital
460 West Oak St. 71730
501 863-2266

FORT SMITH
St. Edward's Mercy
Medical Center
7301 Rogers Ave. 72903
501 452-5100   Ext. 2043

Sparks Regional Med. Ctr.
1311 S. Eye St. 72901
501 441-5011

HARRISON
Boone County Hospital
620 N. Willow St. 72601
501 741-6141   Ext. 275, 276

HELENA
Helena Hospital
Newman Drive
72342
501 338-6411   Ext. 340

LITTLE ROCK
Univ. of Arkansas
Medical Center
4301 W. Markham St. 72201
501 661-6161

OSCEOLA
Osceola Memorial Hosp.
611 Lee Avenue, West
72370
501 563-7180

PINE BLUFF
Jefferson Hospital
1515 W. 42nd Ave.
71601
501 535-6800   Ext. 4706

CALIFORNIA

STATE
COORDINATOR
916 322-2300

Department of Health
Sacramento 95814

FRESNO
Central Valley Regional
Poison Control Ctr.
Fresno Community Hospital
& Medical Center
Fresno & R. Streets
P.O. Box 1232 93715
209 445-1222

LOS ANGELES
Thos. J. Fleming Memorial
Center
Children's Hospital of
Los Angeles
P.O. Box 54700
4650 Sunset Blvd. 90054
213 664-2121

OAKLAND
Children's Hosp. of the
East Bay
51st & Grove Sts.
94609
415 654-5600   Ext. 343

ORANGE
University of California
Irvine Medical Center
101 City Drive South
92688
714 634-5988
634-6011

*SACRAMENTO
Sacramento Medical Center
2315 Stockton Blvd.
95817
916 453-3692
800 852-7221

*SAN DIEGO
San Diego Poison Information
Center
University Hospital
225 W. Dickinson St.
92103
714 294-6000

SAN FRANCISCO
San Francisco General Hosp.
1001 Potrerro Avenue
94102
415 666-2845
800 792-0720

SAN JOSE
Santa Clara Valley
Medical Center
751 S. Bascom Avenue
95128
408 279-5112   Ext. 318, 319

COLORADO

STATE
COORDINATOR
303 320-8476

Department of Health; EMS Division
Denver 80220

DENVER
Rocky Mt. Poison Center
West 8th & Cherokee
80204
303 629-1123

CONNECTICUT

STATE
COORDINATOR
203 674-3456

University of Connecticut Health Center
Farmington 06032

BRIDGEPORT
Bridgeport Hospital
267 Grant St. 06610
203 384-3566

St. Vincent's Hospital
2820 Main St. 06606
203 576-5178

*AAPCC Designated Regional Center

DANBURY
Danbury Hospital
95 Locust Ave. 06810
203 797-7300

FARMINGTON
Connecticut Poison Center
University of Connecticut
Health Center 06032
203 674-3456

MIDDLETOWN
Middlesex Memorial Hosp.
28 Crescent St. 06457
203 347-9471

NEW HAVEN
The Hosp. of St. Raphael
1450 Chapel St. 06511
203 789-3464

Drug Information Center
Dept. of Pharm. Serv.
Yale–New Haven Hospital
789 Howard Ave. 06504
203 436-1960

NORWALK
Norwalk Hospital
24 Stevens St. 06852
203 852-2160

WATERBURY
St. Mary's Hospital
56 Franklin Street 06702
203 574-6011

DELAWARE

WILMINGTON
Wilmington Medical Center
Delaware Division
501 W. 14th Street
19899
302 655-3389

DISTRICT OF COLUMBIA

STATE
COORDINATOR
202 673-6694

Department of Human Services
Washington, DC 20009

WASHINGTON, DC
Children's Hospital National
Medical Center
111 Michigan Avenue, N.W.
20010
202 745-2000

*WASHINGTON, DC
National Capitol Poison
Center
Georgetown Univ. Hosp.
3800 Reservoir Rd. 20007

*Scheduled to become operational October 1, 1980

FLORIDA

STATE
COORDINATOR
904 487-1566

Department of Health and
Rehabilitative Services
Tallahassee 32301

APALACHICOLA
George E. Weems Mem.
Hosp. P.O. Box 610
Franklin Square 32320
904 653-8853

BARTOW
Polk General Hospital
2010 E. Georgia St.
P.O. Box 81 33830
813 533-1111   Ext. 204–237

BRADENTON
Manatee Memorial Hosp.
206 2nd St. E. 33505
813 746-5111   Ext. 466

DAYTONA BEACH
Halifax Hospital
Dept. of Emerg. Serv.
P.O. Box 1990 32014
904 258-1515

FT. LAUDERDALE
Broward General Med. Ctr.
1600 S. Andrews Ave.
33316
305 463-3131   Ext. 1511

FORT MYERS
Lee Memorial Hospital
2776 Cleveland Ave.
P.O. Drawer 2218 33902
813 332-1111   Ext. 285

FT. WALTON BEACH
General Hospital of
Ft. Walton Beach
1000 Mar-Walt Drive
32548
904 242-1111   Ext. 106

GAINESVILLE
Shands Teaching Hosp.
and Clinics
University of Florida
32610
904 392-3746

INVERNESS
Citrus Memorial Hospital
502 Highland Blvd.
32650
904 726-1551

JACKSONVILLE
St. Vincent's Med. Ctr.
Barrs & Johns Ave.
32204
904 389-7751   Ext. 8315

KEY WEST
Florida Keys Mem. Hosp.
600 Junior College Rd.
Stock Island 33040
305 294-5531

LAKELAND
Lakeland General Hosp.
Lakeland Hills Blvd.
P.O. Box 480 33802
813 686-4913

LEESBURG
  Leesburg General Hosp.
  600 E. Dixie 32748
904 787-7222   Ext. 381

MELBOURNE
  James E. Holmes Regional
    Medical Center
  1350 S. Hickory St.
  32901
305 727-7000   Ext. 675

MIAMI
  Jackson Memorial Hosp.
  Att: Pharmacy
  1611 N.W. 12th Ave. 33136
305 325-6799

NAPLES
  Naples Community Hosp.
  350 7th St. N. 33940
813 262-3131   Ext. 2221

NORTH MIAMI BEACH
  Parkway General
    Hospital, Inc.
  160 Northwest 170th St.
  33169
305 651-1100

OCALA
  Munroe Memorial Hosp.
  140 S.E. Orange St.
  P.O. Box 6000
  32670
904 732-1111   Ext. 187

ORLANDO
  Orlando Reg. Med. Ctr.
  Orange Memorial Division
  1414 S. Kuhl Avenue
  32806
305 841-5222

PANAMA CITY
  Bay Memorial Med. Ctr.
  600 N. MacArthur Ave.
  32401
904 769-1511   Ext. 415–416

PENSACOLA
  Baptist Hospital
  1000 W. Moreno St.
  32501
904 434-4811

PUNTA GORDA
  Medical Center Hospital
  809 E. Marion Avenue
  33950
813 639-3131

GUAM

STATE   Guam Memorial Hospital
COORDINATOR   P.O. BOX AX
646-5801   Agana 96910

AGANA
  Pharmacy Service, Box 7696
  U.S. Naval Regional Medical
    Center (GUAM)
  FPO San Francisco, CA 96630
671 344-9265
    344-9354

HAWAII

STATE   Department of Health
COORDINATOR   Honolulu 96801
808 531-7776

HONOLULU
    Kapiolani-Children's
    Medical Center
    1319 Punahou St. 96826
808 941-4411

IDAHO

STATE   Department of Health and Welfare
COORDINATOR   Boise 83701
208 334-2241
TOLL-FREE-STATEWIDE # 1-800 632-8000

BOISE
    St. Alphonsus Hospital
    1055 N. Curtis Rd.
    83704
208 376-1211   Ext. 707

POCATELLO
    St. Anthony Hospital
    650 North 7th Street
    83201
208 232-2733   Ext. 244

IDAHO FALLS
    Idaho Falls Hospital
    Emergency Department
    900 Memorial Dr. 83401
208 529-6111

ILLINOIS

STATE   Division of Emergency Medical Services
COORDINATOR   and Highway Safety
217 785-2080   Springfield 62761

Poison Information & Treatment

Chicago Area Poison Resource Center

CHICAGO
    Rush-Presbyterian-St. Lukes
    Medical Center
    1753 West Congress Parkway
    60612
(312) 942-5969

Northern and Central Poison Resource Center

PEORIA
St. Francis Hospital &
Medical Center
530 N.E. Glen Oak Avenue
61637
(309) 672-2334
1-800 322-5330 (TOLL FREE)

Central and Southern Poison Resource Center

SPRINGFIELD
St. John's Hospital
800 East Carpenter
62702
(217) 753-3330
1-800 252-2022 (TOLL FREE)

INDIANA

STATE   State Board of Health
COORDINATOR   Indianapolis 46206
317 633-0332

ANDERSON
Community Hospital
1515 N. Madison Ave.
46012
317 646-5198

St. John's Hickey
Memorial Hospital
2015 Jackson St.
46014
317 646-8251

ANGOLA
Cameron Memorial
Hospital, Inc.
416 East Maumee St.
46703
219 665-2141   Ext. 146

COLUMBUS
Bartholomew County Hosp.
2400 East 17th St.
47201
812 376-5277

CROWN POINT
St. Anthony Med. Ctr.
Main at Franciscan Rd.
46307
219 738-2100

EAST CHICAGO
St. Catherine Hospital
4321 Fir Street
46312
219 392-1700
392-7203

237

ELKHART
  Elkhart General Hosp.
  600 East Blvd. 46514
219 294-2621

EVANSVILLE
  Deaconess Hospital
  600 Mary St. 47710
812 426-3405

  St. Mary's Hospital
  3700 Washington Ave.
  47715
812 477-6261

  Welborn Memorial
    Baptist Hospital
  401 S.E. 6th St.
  47713
812 426-8000

FORT WAYNE
  Lutheran Hospital
  3024 Fairfield Ave.
  46807
219 458-2211

  Parkview Memorial Hosp.
  220 Randalia Dr.
  46805
219 484-6636   Ext. 7800

  St. Joseph's Hospital
  700 Broadway 46802
219 423-2614

FRANKFORT
  Clinton County Hospital
  1300 S. Jackson St.
  46041
317 654-4451

GARY
  Methodist Hospital of
    Gary, Inc.
  600 Grant Street 46402
219 886-4710

GOSHEN
  Goshen General Hosp.
  200 High Park Avenue
  46526
219 533-2141   Ext. 462

HAMMOND
  St. Margaret Hospital
  25 Douglas Street 46320
219 932-2300   Ext. 700

HUNTINGTON
  Huntington Memorial Hosp.
  1215 Etna Avenue 46750
219 356-3000

INDIANAPOLIS
  Methodist Hospital of
    Indiana, Inc.
  1604 N. Capitol Avenue
  46202
317 927-3033

  Indiana Poison Center
  1001 West 10th Street
  46202
317 630-7351
800 382-9097 (TOLL FREE)

KENDALLVILLE
  McCray Memorial Hospital
  Hospital Drive 46755
219 347-1100

KOKOMO
  Howard Community Hospital
  3500 S. LaFountain Street
  46901
317 453-0702   Ext. 444

LAFAYETTE
  Lafayette Home Hospital
  2400 South Street 47902
317 447-6811

  St. Elizabeth Hospital
  1501 Hartford Street 47904
317 423-6271

LAGRANGE
LaGrange County Hospital
Route #1 46761
219 463-2144

LAPORTE
LaPorte Hospital, Inc.
1007 Lincolnway
46350
219 362-7541   Ext. 212

LEBANON
Witham Memorial Hosp.
1124 N. Lebanon St.
46052
317 482-2700   Ext. 44

MADISON
King's Daughter's Hosp.
112 Presbyterian Ave.
P.O. Box 447 47250
812 265-5211   Ext. 109

MARION
Marion General Hosp.
Wabash & Euclid Ave.
46952
317 662-4694

MISHAWAKA
St. Joseph's Hospital
215 W. 4th St. 46544
219 259-2431

MUNCIE
Ball Memorial Hospital
2401 University Ave.
47303
317 747-3241

PORTLAND
Jay County Hospital
505 W. Arch St.
47371
317 726-7131   Ext. 159

RICHMOND
Reid Memorial Hospital
1401 Chester Blvd.
47374
317 692-7010   Ext. 622

SHELBYVILLE
Wm. S. Major Hospital
150 W. Washington St.
46176
317 392-3211   Ext. 52

SOUTH BEND
St. Joseph's Hospital
811 E. Madison St.
46622
219 234-2151   Ext. 253, 264

TERRE HAUTE
Union Hospital, Inc.
1606 N. 7th St.
47804
812 238-7000   Ext. 7523

VALPARAISO
Porter Memorial Hosp.
814 LaPorte Ave.
46383
219 464-8611   Ext. 232, 312, 334

VINCENNES
The Good Samaritan
Hospital
520 S. 7th St. 47591
812 885-3348

IOWA

STATE
COORDINATOR
515 281-4964

Department of Health
Des Moines 50319

DES MOINES
Iowa Methodist Hosp.
(Blank Memorial Hosp.)
1200 Pleasant Street
50308
515 283-6212

IOWA CITY
Univ. of Iowa Hosp.
Poison Information Center
52240
319 356-1616
800 272-6477 (All Iowa Residents)

DUBUQUE
Mercy Medical Center
Mercy Drive 52001
319 588-8210

WATERLOO
Allen Memorial Hosp.
1825 Logan Avenue
50703
319 235-3941

FORT DODGE
Trinity Regional Hosp.
Poison Information Center
Kenyon Rd. 50501
515 573-3101

KANSAS

STATE
COORDINATOR
913 862-9360
Ext. 542

Kansas Dept. of Health & Environment
Topeka 66620

ATCHISON
Atchison Hospital
1301 N. 2nd St.
66002
913 367-2131

EMPORIA
Newman Memorial Hosp.
12th & Chestnut Streets
66801
316 343-6800   Ext. 545

DODGE CITY
Dodge City Reg. Hosp.
Ross & Ave. "A"
P.O. Box 1478
67801
316 225-2036

FORT RILEY
Irwin Army Hospital
66442
913 239-7776

FORT SCOTT
Mercy Hospital
821 Burke St.
66701
316 223-2200   Night: 223-0476

GREAT BEND
Central Kansas
Medical Center
3515 Broadway
67530
316 793-3523   Night: 792-2511

HAYS
Hadley Regional
Medical Center
201 E. 7th St.
67601
913 628-8251

KANSAS CITY
Univ. of Kansas
Medical Center
39th & Rainbow Blvd.
66103
913 588-6633

Bethany Medical Ctr.
51 No. 12th St.
66102
913 281-8880

LAWRENCE
Lawrence Memorial Hosp.
325 Maine St. 66044
913 843-3680   Ext. 162, 163

PARSONS
Labette County
Medical Center
S. 21st St. 67357
316 421-4880   Ext. 320

SALINA
St. John's Hospital
139 N. Penn St.
67401
913 827-5591   Ext. 112

TOPEKA
Stormont-Vail Regional
Medical Center
10th & Washburn Sts.
66606
913 354-6100

WICHITA
Wesley Medical Ctr.
550 N. Hillside Ave.
67214
316 685-2151   Ext. 7515

KENTUCKY

STATE
COORDINATOR
502 564-4935

Department for Human Resources
Frankfort 40601

ASHLAND
King's Daughters Hosp.
2201 Lexington Ave.
41101
606 324-2222

BEREA
Porter Moore Drug, Inc.
124 Main St. 40403
606 986-3061

FORT THOMAS
St. Lukes Hospital
85 N. Grand Ave. 41075
606 292-3215

LEXINGTON
Central Baptist Hosp.
1740 S. Limestone St.
40503
606 278-3411

Drug Information Ctr.
University of Kentucky
Medical Ctr. 40536
606 233-5320

LOUISVILLE
Norton-Children's Hosp.
Pharmacy Dept.
200 E. Chestnut St.
40202
502 589-8222

MURRAY
Murray-Calloway
County Hospital
803 Popular 42071
502 753-7588

OWENSBORO
Owensboro-Daviess
County Hospital
811 Hospital Court
42301
502 926-3030   Ext. 180, 174
(24 Hours)

PADUCAH
Western Baptist Hosp.
2501 Kentucky Ave.
42001
502 444-6361   Ext. 105
Night: 199

PRESTONSBURG
Poison Control Center
Highlands Reg. Med. Ctr.
41653
606 886-8511   Ext. 160

SOUTH WILLIAMSON
Appalachian Reg. Hosp.
Central Pharmaceutical
Service
2000 Central Ave. 25661
606 237-5686

LOUISIANA

STATE
COORDINATOR
504 342-2600

Bureau of Emergency Medical Services
Baton Rouge 70801

ALEXANDRIA
Rapides General Hosp.
Emergency Dept.
P.O. Box 7146 71301
318 487-8111

BATON ROUGE
Doctors Hospital
2414 Bunker Hill Dr.
70808
504 927-9050

LAFAYETTE
Our Lady of Lourdes Hosp.
P.O. Box 3827
611 St. Landry St. 70501
318 234-7381

LAKE CHARLES
Lake Charles Memorial
Hospital
P.O. Drawer M 70601
318 478-6800

MONROE
School of Pharmacy
Northeast Louisiana Univ.
700 University Avenue
71209
218 342-2008

St. Francis Hospital
P.O. Box 1901 71301
318 325-6454

NEW ORLEANS
Charity Hosp. of New Orleans
1532 Tulane Avenue
70140
504 568-5222

SHREVEPORT
LSU Medical Center
P.O. Box 33932 71130
318 425-1524

MAINE

STATE
COORDINATOR
1-800 442-6305

Maine Poison Control Center
Portland 04102

PORTLAND
Maine Medical Center
22 Bramhall Street
04102
207 871-2950
1-800 442-6305

MARYLAND

STATE
COORDINATOR
301 728-7604

Maryland Poison Information Center
University of Maryland School of Pharmacy
21201

BALTIMORE
Maryland Poison Inf. Ctr.
Univ. of MD. Sch. of Ph.
636 W. Lombard St. 21201
301 528-7701
800 492-2414
(TOLL FREE in MARYLAND)

CUMBERLAND
Sacred Heart Hospital
900 Seton Drive
21502
301 722-6677

MASSACHUSETTS

STATE Department of Public Health
COORDINATOR Boston 02111
617 727-2670

*BOSTON
Massachusetts Poison
  Control System
300 Longwood Avenue
02115
617 232-2120
1-800 682-9211 (TOLL FREE)

MICHIGAN

STATE Department of Public Health
COORDINATOR Lansing 48909
517 373-1406

ADRIAN
  Emma L. Bixby Hosp.
  818 Riverside Ave.
  49221
517 263-2412

ANN ARBOR
  University Hospital
  1405 E. Ann St.
  48104
313 764-5102

BATTLE CREEK
  Community Hospital
  183 West St.
  49016
616 963-5521

BAY CITY
  Bay Medical Center
  100 15th St.
  48706
517 892-6589

BERRIEN CENTER
  Berrien General Hosp.
  Dean's Hill Rd.
  49102
616 471-7761

COLDWATER
  Community Health Ctr.
  of Branch County
  274 E. Chicago St.
  49036
517 278-7361

*DETROIT
  Children's Hospital
  of Michigan
  Southeast Regional Poison
  Center
  3901 Beaubien 48201
313 494-5711

AAPCC Designated Regional Center

Mount Carmel Mercy
Hospital
6071 W. Outer Dr.
48235
313 864-5400   Ext. 416

ELOISE
Wayne County General
Hospital
30712 Michigan Avenue
48132
Day: 313 722-3748
Night: 274-3000-6231

FLINT
Hurley Hospital
6th Ave. & Begole
48502
313 766-0111

GRAND RAPIDS
St. Mary's Hospital
201 Lafayette, S.E.
49503
616 774-6794

Western Michigan Regional
Poison Center
1840 Wealthy, S.E.
49506
*800 442-4571
800 632-2727 (TOLL FREE)

HANCOCK
Portage View Hospital
200–210 Michigan Ave.
49930
906 492-1122   Ext. 209

HOLLAND
Holland Community Hosp.
602 Michigan Ave.
49423
616 396-4661

JACKSON
W.A. Foote Memorial
Hospital
205 N. East St.
49201
517 788-4816

KALAMAZOO
Midwest Poison Ctr.
Borgess Medical Ctr.
1521 Gull Rd. 49001
616 383-4815

Bronson Methodist Hosp.
252 E. Lovell St.
49006
616 383-6409

LANSING
St. Lawrence Hospital
1210 W. Saginaw St.
48914
517 372-5112
372-5113

MARQUETTE
Marquette General Hosp.
Upper Peninsula Regional
Poison Center
420 W. Magnetic Dr. 49855
800 562-9723

MIDLAND
Midland Hospital
4005 Orchard Dr.
48640
517 631-7700   Ext. 304

PETOSKEY
Little Traverse Hosp.
416 Connable
49770
616 347-7373

PONTIAC
St. Joseph Mercy Hosp.
900 Woodward Avenue
48053
313 858-7373
858-7374

PORT HURON
Port Huron Hospital
1001 Kearney St.
48060
313 987-5555
987-5000

SAGINAW
Saginaw General Hosp.
1447 N. Harrison
48602
517 755-1111

TRAVERSE CITY
Munson Medical Ctr.
Sixth St. 49684
616 947-6140

MINNESOTA

STATE COORDINATOR
612 296-5281

State Department of Health
Minneapolis 55404

BEMIDJI
Bemidji Hospital
56601
218 751-5430

BRAINERD
St. Joseph's Hospital
56401
218 829-2861   Ext. 211

CROOKSTON
Riverview Hospital
320 S. Hubbard
56716
218 281-4682

DULUTH
St. Luke's Hospital
Emergency Department
915 E. First St. 55805
218 727-6636

St. Mary's Hospital
407 E. 3rd St. 55805
218 727-4551   Ext. 359

EDINA
Fairview-Southdale Hosp.
6401 France Ave., S.
55435
612 920-4400

FERGUS FALLS
Lake Region Hospital
56537
218 736-5475

FRIDLEY
Unity Hospital
550 Osborne Rd. 55432
612 786-2200

MANKATO
Immanuel-St. Joseph's
Hospital
325 Garden Blvd. 56001
507 387-4031

MARSHALL
Louis Weiner Memorial
Hospital 56258
507 532-9661

MINNEAPOLIS
   Fairview Hospital
   Outpatient Department
   2312 S. 6th St. 55406
612 371-6402

   Hennepin Poison Center
   Hennepin County Med. Ctr.
   701 Park Ave. 55415
*612 347-3141
**

MINNEAPOLIS
   North Memorial Hospital
   3220 Lowry North 55422
612 588-0616

   Northwestern Hospital
   810 E. 27th St. 55407
612 874-4233

MORRIS
   Stevens County Memorial
      Hospital 56267
612 589-1313

ROCHESTER
   Southeastern Minnesota
      Poison Control Center
   St. Mary's Hospital
   1216 Second St., S.W.
   55901
507 285-5123

ST. CLOUD
   St. Cloud Hospital
   1406 6th Avenue, N.
   56301
612 251-2700   Ext. 221

ST. PAUL
   Bethesda Lutheran Hosp.
   559 Capitol Blvd. 55103
612 221-2301

   The Children's Hosp. Inc.
   311 Pleasant Ave. 55102
612 227-6521

   St. John's Hospital
   403 Maria Ave. 55106
612 228-3132

   St. Joseph's Hospital
   69 W. Exchange 55102
612 291-3348
   291-3139

   United Hospitals, Inc.
   St. Luke's Division
   300 Pleasant Ave. 55102
612 298-8402

   St. Paul-Ramsey Hosp.
   640 Jackson St. 55101
612 221-2113

WILLMAR
   Rice Memorial Hospital
   402 W. 3rd St. 56201
612 235-4543

WORTHINGTON
   Worthington Regional
      Hospital
   1016 6th Ave. 56187
507 372-2941

---

*AAPCC Designated Center
**Receives State grant to provide 24-hour TOLL FREE telephone information service to all
State residents.

MISSISSIPPI

STATE
COORDINATOR
601 354-6650

State Board of Health
Jackson 39205

BILOXI
Gulf Coast Community Hosp.
4642 West Beach Blvd.
39531
601 388-1919

USAF Hospital Keesler
Keesler Air Force Base
39534
601 377-2516
377-6555
377-6556

BRANDON
Rankin General Hospital
350 Crossgates Blvd.
39042
601 825-2811   Ext. 487, 488

COLUMBIA
Marion County General
Hospital
39429
601 736-6303   Ext. 217

GREENWOOD
Greenwood-Leflore
Hospital
River Road 38930
601 453-9751   Ext. 2633

HATTIESBURG
Forrest County General
Hospital
400 S. 28th Ave. 39401
601 264-4235

JACKSON
Mississippi Baptist
Medical Center
1225 N. State St.
39201
601 968-1704

St. Dominic–Jackson
Memorial Hospital
969 Lakeland Dr.
39216
601 982-0121   Ext. 2345, 2346,
2347

State Board of Health
Bureau of Disease
Control 39205
601 354-6650

University Medical Center
2500 N. State Street
39216
601 354-7660

LAUREL
Jones County Community
Hospital
Jefferson St. at 13th Ave.
39440
601 649-4000   Ext. 207, 218, 220,
248

MERIDIAN
Meridian Regional Hosp.
Highway 39, North
39301
601 483-6211   Ext. 54, 71

PASCAGOULA
Singing River Hospital
Highway 90 East
39567
601 938-5162

UNIVERSITY
School of Pharmacy
University of
Mississippi 38677
601 234-1522

VICKSBURG
Mercy Regional Medical
Center
100 McAuley Dr. 39181
601 636-2131   Ext. 250, 251, 276

MISSOURI

STATE
COORDINATOR
314 751-2713

Missouri Division of Health
Jefferson City 65102

CAPE GIRARDEAU
St. Francis Medical Ctr.
St. Francis Drive
63701
314 335-1251   Ext. 217

COLUMBIA
University of Missouri
Medical Center
807 Stadium Rd. 65201
314 882-4141

HANNIBAL
St. Elizabeth's Hospital
109 Virginia St.
63401
314 221-0414   Ext. 101, 183

JEFFERSON CITY
Charles E. Still
Osteopathic Hosp.
1125 S. Madison 65101
314 635-7141   Ext. 215

JOPLIN
St. John's Medical Ctr.
2727 McClelland Blvd.
64801
417 781-2727   Ext. 393

*KANSAS CITY
Children's Mercy Hosp.
24th at Gillham Rd.
64108
816 234-3000

KIRKSVILLE
Kirksville Osteopathic
Hospital
800 W. Jefferson St.
63501
816 626-2266

POPLAR BLUFF
Lucy Lee Hospital
330 N. 2nd St.
63901
314 785-7721

*AAPCC Designated Regional Center

ROLLA
Phelps County Memorial
Hospital
1000 W. 10th St.
65401
314 364-3100   Ext. 136, 137

ST. JOSEPH
Methodist Medical Ctr.
Seventh to Ninth on
Faraon Street
64501
816 271-7580
232-8481

*ST. LOUIS
Cardinal Glennon Memorial
Hospital for Children
1465 S. Grand Boulevard
63104
314 772-5200

St. Louis Children's
Hospital
500 S. Kingshighway
63110
314 367-2034

SPRINGFIELD
Lester E. Cox Medical Ctr.
1423 N. Jefferson St.
65802
417 831-9746
1-800 492-4824 (TOLL FREE)

St. John's Hospital
1235 E. Cherokee
65802
417 885-2115

WEST PLAINS
West Plains Memorial
Hospital
1103 Alaska Avenue
65775
417 256-9111   Ext. 258, 259

MONTANA

STATE   Department of Health and Environmental Sciences
COORDINATOR   Helena 59601
1-800 525-5042

Montana Poison Control
System
1-800 525-5042 (TOLL FREE)

*AAPCC Designated Regional Center

NEBRASKA

STATE   Department of Health
COORDINATOR   Lincoln 68502
402 471-2122

*OMAHA
   Children's Memorial Hosp.
   44th & Dewey Sts.
   68105
402 553-5400
800 642-9999 (NEBRASKA)
800 228-9515
   (SURROUNDING STATES)

NEVADA

STATE   Department of Human Resources
COORDINATOR   Carson City 89710
702 885-4750

LAS VEGAS
   Southern Nevada Memorial
     Hospital
   1800 W. Charleston Blvd.
   89102
702 385-1277

   Sunrise Hospital Med. Ctr.
   3186 South Maryland Parkway
   89109
702 731-8000

RENO
   St. Mary's Hospital
   235 W. 6th 89503
702 323-2041

   Washoe Medical Center
   77 Pringle Way 89502
702 785-4129
Night: 785-4140

NEW HAMPSHIRE

HANOVER
   New Hampshire Poison Center
   Mary Hitchcock Hospital
   2 Maynard St. 03755
603 643-4000

---

*AAPCC Designated Regional Center

NEW JERSEY

STATE Department of Health
COORDINATOR Trenton 08625
609 292-5666

ATLANTIC CITY
Atlantic City Medical
Center
1925 Pacific Ave.
08401
609 344-4081

BELLEVILLE
Clara Maass Memorial
Hospital
1A Franklin Ave.
07109
201 751-1000   Ext. 781, 782, 783

BOONTON
Riverside Hospital
Powerville Rd.
07055
201 334-5000   Ext. 186, 187

BRIDGETON
Bridgeton Hospital
Irving Ave. 08302
609 451-6600

CAMDEN
West Jersey Hospital
Evesham Ave. and
    Voorhees Twp. 08104
609 795-5554

DENVILLE
St. Clare's Hospital
Pocono Rd. 07834
201 627-3000   Ext. 6063

EAST ORANGE
East Orange General
Hospital
300 Central Ave.
07019
201 672-8400   Ext. 223

ELIZABETH
St. Elizabeth Hosp.
225 Williamson St.
07207
201 527-5059

ENGLEWOOD
Englewood Hospital
350 Engle Street
07631
201 894-3262

FLEMINGTON
Hunterdon Medical Ctr.
Route #31 08822
201 782-2121

LIVINGSTON
St. Barnabas Medical
Center
Old Short Hills Rd.
07039
201 922-5161

LONG BRANCH
Monmouth Medical Ctr.
Dunbar & 2nd Ave.
07740
201 222-2210

MONTCLAIR
Mountainside Hospital
Bay & Highland Aves.
07042
201 746-6000

MOUNT HOLLY
Burlington County
Memorial Hosp.
175 Madison Ave.
08060
609 267-7877

NEPTUNE
Jersey Shore Medical
Ctr.-Fitkin Hosp.
1945 Corlies Ave.
07753
800 822-9761

NEWARK
Newark Beth Israel
Medical Center
201 Lyons Ave.
07112
201 926-7240
926-7241,
926-7243

NEW BRUNSWICK
Middlesex General Hosp.
180 Somerset Street
08903
201 828-3000   Ext. 425, 308

St. Peter's Medical Ctr.
254 Easton Ave. 08903
201 745-8527

NEWTON
Newton Memorial Hosp.
175 High St. 07860
201 383-2121   Ext. 270, 1, 2,
273

ORANGE
Hospital Center at
Orange
188 S. Essex Ave.
07051
201 266-2120

PASSAIC
St. Mary's Hospital
211 Pennington Ave.
07055
201 473-1000   Ext. 441

PERTH AMBOY
Perth Amboy General Hosp.
530 New Brunswick Ave.
08861
201 442-3700   Ext. 2500

PHILLIPSBURG
Warren Hospital
185 Roseberry St.
08865
201 859-1500   Ext. 280

POINT PLEASANT
Point Pleasant Hosp.
Osborn Ave. & River
Front 08742
201 892-1100   Ext. 385

PRINCETON
The Medical Center at
Princeton
253 Witherspoon St.
08540
609 734-4554

SADDLE BROOK
Saddle Brook General
Hospital
300 Market St. 07662
201 368-6026

SOMERS POINT
    Shore Memorial Hosp.
    Brighton & Sunny Aves.
    08244
609 653-3515

SOMERVILLE
    Somerset Medical Center
    Rehill Ave. 08876
201 725-4000   Ext. 431, 432, 433

SUMMIT
    Overlook Hospital
    193 Morris Ave.
    07901
201 522-2232

TEANECK
    Holy Name Hospital
    718 Teaneck Rd.
    07666
201 833-3000

TRENTON
    Helene Fuld Med. Ctr.
    750 Brunswick Ave.
    08638
609 396-1077

UNION
    Memorial General Hosp.
    1000 Galloping Hill Rd.
    07083
201 687-1900   Ext. 237

WAYNE
    Greater Paterson Gen.
    Hospital
    224 Hamburg Tnpk.
    07470
201 942-6900   Ext. 224, 225, 226

NEW MEXICO

STATE   The University of New Mexico
COORDINATOR   Albuquerque, 87131
505 843-2551

*STATE COORDINATOR
ALBUQUERQUE
    New Mexico Poison,
        Drug Inf. & Med.
        Crisis Ctr., Univ.
        of New Mexico 87131
505 843-2551
(1-800 432-6866 Within NM)

---

*AAPCC Designated Regional Center

NEW YORK

STATE — Department of Health
COORDINATOR — Albany 12210
518 474-3785

BINGHAMTON
Southern Tier Poison Ctr.
Binghamton General Hosp.
Mitchell Avenue
13903
607 723-8929

Our Lady of Lourdes
Memorial Hosp.
169 Riverside Drive
13905
607 798-5231

BUFFALO
Western NY Poison Control
Center
Children's Hospital
219 Bryant St. 14222
716 878-7000
878-7654
878-7655

DUNKIRK
Brooks Memorial Hosp.
10 West 6th St.
14048
716 366-1111   Ext. 414, 415

*EAST MEADOW
Long Island Poison Ctr. at
Nassau County Medical Ctr.
2201 Hempstead Tnpk.
11554
516 542-2323
542-2324
542-2325

ELMIRA
Arnot Ogden Memorial
Hospital
Roe Ave. & Grove Street
14901
607 737-4100

St. Joseph's Hospital
Health Center
555 E. Market St.
14901
607 734-2662

ENDICOTT
Ideal Hospital
600 High Street
13760
607 754-7171

GLENS FALLS
Glens Falls Hospital
100 Park St. 12801
518 792-3151   Ext. 456

JAMESTOWN
W.C.A. Hospital
207 Foote Ave.
14701
716 487-0141
484-8648

JOHNSON CITY
Wilson Memorial Hosp.
33–57 Harrison St.
14707
607 773-6611

---

*AAPCC Designated Regional Center

KINGSTON
Kingston Hospital
396 Broadway
12401
914 331-3131

NEW YORK
N.Y. City Poison Control
Center
Department of Hlth., Bureau of
Laboratories
455 First Avenue 10016
212 340-4494
340-4495

NYACK
Hudson Valley Poison Center
Nyack Hospital
North Midland Avenue
10960
914 358-6200   Ext. 451, 452

*ROCHESTER
Finger Lakes Poison Control Ctr.
LIFE LINE, Univ. of Rochester
Medical Center 14620
716 275-5151

SCHENECTADY
Ellis Hospital
1101 Nott Street
12308
518 382-4039
382-4121

SYRACUSE
Syracuse Poison Information
Ctr.
Upstate Medical Ctr.
750 E. Adams Street
13210
315 476-7529
473-5831

TROY
St. Mary's Hospital
1300 Massachusetts Ave.
12180
518 272-5792

UTICA
St. Luke's Hospital Ctr.
P.O. Box 479
13502
315 798-6200

WATERTOWN
House of the Good
Samaritan Hospital
Washington & Pratt Sts. 13602
315 788-8700

NORTH CAROLINA

STATE Duke University Medical Center
COORDINATOR Durham 27710
919 684-8111

*AAPCC Designated Regional Center

ASHEVILLE
Western N.C. Poison
Control Center
Memorial Mission Hosp.
509 Biltmore Avenue
28801
704 255-4660

CHARLOTTE
Mercy Hospital
2001 Vail Ave. 28207
704 379-5827

DURHAM
Duke University
Medical Center
Box 3007 27710
919 684-8111

GREENSBORO
Moses Cone Hospital
1200 N. Elm St. 27420
919 379-4105

HENDERSONVILLE
Margaret R. Pardee
Memorial Hospital
Fleming St. 28739
704 693-6522   Ext. 555, 556

HICKORY
Catawba Memorial Hosp.
Fairgrove-Church Rd.
28601
704 322-6649

JACKSONVILLE
Onslow Memorial Hosp.
Western Blvd.
28540
919 353-7610   Ext. 240

WILMINGTON
New Hanover Memorial
Hospital
2131 S. 17th St. 28401
919 343-7046

NORTH DAKOTA

STATE
COORDINATOR
701 224-2388

Department of Health
Bismarck 58505

BISMARCK
Bismarck Hospital
300 North 7th St.
58501
701 223-4357

FARGO
St. Luke's Hospital
Fifth St. at Mills Ave.
58122
701 280-5575

GRAND FORKS
United Hospital
1200 S. Columbia Rd.
58201
701 780-5000

MINOT
St. Joseph's Hospital
Third St. & Fourth Ave., S.E.
58701
701 857-2553

WILLISTON
Mercy Hospital
1301 15th Avenue, W.
58801
701 572-7661

OHIO

STATE   Department of Health
COORDINATOR   Columbus 43216
614 466-2544

AKRON
    Children's Hospital
    281 Locust
    44308
216 379-8562

CANTON
    Aultman Hospital
    Emergency Rm.
    2600 Sixth Street S.W.
    44710
216 452-9911   Ext. 203

CINCINNATI
    Drug & Poison Inf. Ctr.
    Univ. of Cincinnati Med.
    Ctr., Room 7701, Bridge
    45267
513 872-5111

CLEVELAND
    Academy of Medicine
    11001 Cedar Avenue
    44106
216 231-8082

COLUMBUS
    Children's Hospital
    700 Children's Dr.
    43205
614 228-1323

DAYTON
    Children's Medical Ctr.
    One Children's Plaza
    45404
513 222-2227

LORAIN
    Lorain Community Hosp.
    3700 Kolbe Rd. 44053
216 282-2220

MANSFIELD
    Mansfield General Hosp.
    335 Glessner Ave.
    44903
419 522-3411   Ext. 545

SPRINGFIELD
    Community Hospital
    2615 E. High St.
    45505
513 325-1255

TOLEDO
    Poison Information Center
    Medical College Hospital
    P.O. Box 6190 43609
419 381-3897
10008 (Caller Service)

YOUNGSTOWN
    Mahoning Valley Poison
    Center
    St. Eliz. Hosp. & Med. Ctr.
    1044 Belmont Avenue 44505
216 746-2222

ZANESVILLE
    Bethesda Hospital
    Poison Information Center
    2951 Maple Avenue 43701
614 454-4221

OKLAHOMA

STATE
COORDINATOR
405 271-5454
or
800 522-4611

Oklahoma Poison Control Center
Oklahoma Children's Memorial Hospital
P.O. Box 26307
63126

ADA
Valley View Hospital
1300 E. 6th St.
74820
405 322-2323   Ext. 200

ARDMORE
Memorial Hospital of
Southern Oklahoma
1011-14th Ave. 73401
405 223-5400

LAWTON
Comanche County
Memorial Hosp.
3401 Gore Blvd. 73501
405 355-8620

McALESTER
McAlester General
Hosp., Inc. West
P.O. Box 669 74501
918 426-1800   Ext. 240

OKLAHOMA CITY
Oklahoma Poison Control
Center
Oklahoma Children's
Memorial Hospital
P.O. Box 26307 73126
405 271-5454
or
800 522-4611 (Oklahoma)

PONCA CITY
St. Joseph Medical Ctr.
14th & Hartford 74601
405 765-3321

TULSA
Hillcrest Medical Ctr.
1653 East 12th
74104
918 584-1351   Ext. 6165

OREGON

PORTLAND
Oregon Poison Control &
Drug Inf. Center
Univ. of Oregon Hlth.
Sciences Center
3181 S.W. Sam Jackson
Park Road 97201
503 225-8968
1-800 452-7165

PANAMA

ANCON
    U.S.A. MEDDAC Panama
    ATTN: Gorgas US Army
      Hospital
    APO Miami 34004
507 52-7500

PENNSYLVANIA

        STATE   Department of Health
        COORDINATOR Harrisburg 17120
        717 787-2307

ALLENTOWN
    Lehigh Valley Poison
      Center
    17th & Chew Sts. 18103
215 433-2311

ALTOONA
    Altoona Region Poison
      Center, Mercy Hospital
    2500 Seventh Ave. 16603
814 946-3711

BETHLEHEM
    St. Luke's Hospital
    800 Ostrum St. 18015
215 691-4141

BLOOMSBURG
    The Bloomsburg Hospital
    549 E. Fair St. 17815
717 784-7121

BRADFORD
    Bradford Hospital
    Interstate Pkwy. 16701
814 368-4143

BRYN MAWR
    The Bryn Mawr Hospital
    19010
215 527-0600

CHAMBERSBURG
    The Chambersburg Hosp.
    7th and King St.
    17201
717 264-5171   Ext. 431

CHESTER
    Sacred Heart General
      Hospital
    9th and Wilson St.
    19013
215 494-0721   Ext. 232

CLEARFIELD
    Clearfield Hospital
    809 Turnpike Ave.
    16830
814 765-5341

COALDALE
Coaldale State General
Hospital 18218
717 645-2131

COUDERSPORT
Charles Cole Memorial
Hospital
RD #3, Route 6 16915
814 274-9300

DANVILLE
Susquehanna Poison
Center
Geisinger Medical Ctr.
North Academy Ave. 17821
717 275-6116

DOYLESTOWN
Doylestown Hospital
595 W. State St. 18901
215 345-2281

DREXEL HILL
Delaware County Memorial
Hospital
Lansdowne & Keystone Ave.
19026
215 259-3800

EAST STROUDSBURG
Pocono Hospital
206 E. Brown St.
18301
717 421-4000

EASTON
Easton Hospital
21st & Lehigh St.
18042
215 250-4000

ERIE
Doctors Osteopathic
252 W. 11th St.
16501
814 455-3961

Erie Osteopathic Hosp.
5515 Peach St. 16509
814 864-4031

Hamot Medical Center
4 E. Second St. 16512
814 455-6711   Ext. 521

Northwest Poison
Center
St. Vincent Health Ctr.
P.O. Box 740 16512
814 452-3232

GETTYSBURG
Annie M. Warner Hosp.
S. Washington St.
17325
717 334-2121

GREENSBURG
Westmoreland Hosp. Assn.
532 W. Pittsburgh St.
15601
412 837-0100

HANOVER
Hanover General Hospital
300 Highland Ave.
17331
717 637-3711

HARRISBURG
Harrisburg Hospital
S. Front & Mulberry St.
17101
717 782-3639

Polyclinic Hospital
3rd & Polyclinic Ave.
17105
717 782-4141   Ext. 4132

HERSHEY
Milton S. Hershey
Medical Center
University Dr. 17033
717 534-6111

JEANNETE
Jeannete District
Memorial Hosp.
600 Jefferson Ave.
15644
412 527-3551

JERSEY SHORE
Jersey Shore Hospital
Thompson St. 17740
717 398-0100

JOHNSTOWN
Conemaugh Valley
Memorial Hosp.
1086 Franklin St.
15905
814 535-5351

Lee Hospital
320 Main St. 15901
814 535-7541

Mercy Hospital
1020 Franklin St. 15905
814 536-5353

LANCASTER
Lancaster General Hosp.
555 North Duke St.
17604
717 299-5511

St. Joseph's Hospital
250 College Ave.
17604
717 299-4546

LANSDALE
North Penn Hospital
7th & Broad St.
19446
215 368-2100

LEBANON
Good Samaritan Hosp.
4th & Walnut Sts.
17042
717 272-7611

LEHIGHTON
Gnaden-Huetten Memorial
Hospital
11th & Hamilton St.
18235
215 377-1300

LEWISTOWN
Lewistown Hospital
Highland Ave. 17044
717 248-5411

MUNCY
Muncy Valley Hospital
P.O. Box 340 17756
717 546-8282

NANTICOKE
Nanticoke State
Hospital
W. Washington St.
18634
717 735-5000

PAOLI
Paoli Memorial Hospital
19301
215 647-2200

PHILADELPHIA
Philadelphia Poison
Information
321 University Avenue
19104
215 922-5523
922-5524

PHILIPSBURG
Philipsburg State
General Hosp.
16866
814 342-3320

PITTSBURGH
Children's Hospital
125 Desoto St. 15213
412 681-6669

PITTSTON
Pittston Hospital
Oregon Heights
18640
717 654-3341

POTTSTOWN
Pottstown Memorial
Medical Ctr.
High St. & Firestone Blvd.
19464
215 327-1000

POTTSVILLE
Good Samaritan Hospital
E. Norwegian and
Tremont St. 17901
717 622-3400

READING
Community General Hosp.
145 N. 6th St. 19601
215 376-4881

Reading Hospital and
Medical Ctr. 19603
215 378-6218

SAYRE
The Robert Packer Hosp.
Guthrie Square 18840
717 888-6666

SELLERSVILLE
Grandview Hospital
18960
215 257-3611

SOMERSET
Somerset Community
Hospital
225 South Center Ave.
15501
814 443-2626

STATE COLLEGE
Centre Community
Hospital 16801
814 238-4351

TITUSVILLE
Titusville Hospital
406 W. Oak St. 16354
814 827-1851

TUNKHANNOCK
Tyler Memorial Hosp.
RD #1 18657
717 836-2161

YORK
Memorial Osteopathic
Hospital
325 S. Belmont St.
17403
717 843-8623

York Hospital
1001 S. George St.
17405
717 771-2311

PUERTO RICO

STATE
COORDINATOR
809 765-4880
765-0615

University of Puerto Rico
Rio Piedras

ARECIBO
District Hospital
of Arecibo 00613
809 878-7272   Ext. 7459, 7510

FAJARDO
District Hospital
of Fajardo 00649
809 863-3792
863-0939

MAYAGUEZ
Mayaguez Medical Ctr.
Department of Health
P.O. Box 1868 00709
809 832-8686   Ext. 1224

PONCE
District Hospital
of Ponce 00731
809 842-8364

RIO PIEDRAS
Medical Center of
Puerto Rico 00936
809 764-3515

SAN JUAN
Pharmacy School
Medical Sciences Campus
GPO Box 5067 00936
809 753-4849 (Information Only)

RHODE ISLAND

STATE
COORDINATOR
401 277-2401

Department of Health
Providence 02908

PROVIDENCE
Rhode Island Hospital
593 Eddy St. 02902
401 277-4000

SOUTH CAROLINA

STATE
COORDINATOR
803 758-5625

Department of Health & Environmental Control
Columbia 29201

CHARLESTON
Poison Information Serv.
Medical University of
South Carolina
171 Ashley Ave. 29403
803 792-4201

COLUMBIA
Palmetto Poison Center
College of Pharmacy
University of South Carolina
29208
803 765-7359
1-800 922-1117 (TOLL FREE)

SOUTH DAKOTA

STATE
COORDINATOR
605 773-3361

Department of Health
Pierre 57501

RAPID CITY
West River Poison Ctr.
Rapid City Regional
Hospital East
57701
605 343-3333
1-800 742-8925 (TOLL FREE)

SIOUX FALLS
McKennan Hospital Poison Ctr.
800 East 21st St.
57101
605 336-3894
1-800 952-0123 (TOLL FREE)

TENNESSEE

STATE
COORDINATOR
615 741-2407

Department of Public Health
Nashville 37219

CHATTANOOGA
T.C. Thompson Children's
Hospital
910 Blackford St. 37403
615 755-6100

JOHNSON CITY
Memorial Hospital
Boone & Fairview Ave.
37601
615 926-1131

COOKEVILLE
Cookeville General Hosp.
142 W. 5th St. 38501
615 528-2541

KNOXVILLE
Memorial Research Center
and Hospital
1924 Alcoa Highway
37920
615 971-3261

JACKSON
Madison General Hosp.
708 W. Forest 38301
901 424-0424

MEMPHIS
Southern Poison Center
University of Tennessee
College of Pharmacy
874 Union Avenue 38163
901 528-6048

NASHVILLE
Vanderbilt University
Hospital
21st & Garland 37232
615 322-3391

TEXAS

STATE
COORDINATOR
512 458-7254

Department of Health Resources
Austin 78756

ABILENE
Hendrick Hospital
19th & Hickory Sts.
79601
915 677-3551   Ext. 266, 267

CORPUS CHRISTI
Memorial Medical Center
P.O. Box 5280
2606 Hospital Blvd.
78405
512 884-4511   Ext. 556, 557

AMARILLO
Amarillo Hospital District
Amarillo Emergency
Receiving Ctr.
P.O. Box 1110
2203 W. 6th St. 79175
806 376-4431   Ext. 501, 502, 503, 504

EL PASO
R.E. Thomason General
Hospital
P.O. Box 20009
4815 Alameda Ave.
79905
915 544-1200

AUSTIN
Brackenridge Hospital
14th & Sabine Sts. 78701
512 478-4490

FORT WORTH
W.I. Cook Children's
Hospital
1212 Lancaster
76102
817 336-5521   Ext. 17
or 336-6611

BEAUMONT
Baptist Hospital of
Southeast Texas
P.O. Box 1591
College & 11th St.
77701
713 833-7409

*GALVESTON
Southeast Texas Poison
Control Center
8th & Mechanic Sts.
77550
713 765-1420

---

*AAPCC Designated Regional Center

HOUSTON
Southeast Texas Poison
Control Center
8th & Mechanic Sts.
Galveston, TX 77550
713 654-1701

HARLINGEN
Valley Baptist Hospital
P.O. Box 2588
2101 S. Commerce St.
78550
512 423-1224   Ext. 283

LAREDO
Mercy Hospital
1515 Logan St.
78040
512 722-2431   Ext. 29

LUBBOCK
Methodist Hospital
Pharmacy
3615 19th St. 79410
806 792-1011   Ext. 315

MIDLAND
Midland Memorial Hospital
1908 W. Wall 79701
915 684-8257

ODESSA
Medical Center Hospital
P.O. Box 633
79760
915 337-7311   Ext. 250, 252

PLAINVIEW
Plainview Hospital
2404 Yonkers St. 79072
806 296-9601

SAN ANGELO
Shannon West Texas
Memorial Hospital
P.O. Box 1879
9 S. Magdalen St.
76901
915 653-6741   Ext. 210

SAN ANTONIO
Department of Pediatrics
Univ. of Texas Health Science
Center at San Antonio
7703 Floyd Curl Dr. 78284
512 223-1481

TYLER
Medical Center Hospital
1000 S. Beckham St.
75701
214 597-0351   Ext. 255

WACO
Hillcrest Baptist Hosp.
3000 Herring Ave.
76708
817 753-1412
756-6111

WICHITA FALLS
Wichita General Hospital
Emergency Room
1600 8th St. 76301
817 322-6771

UTAH

STATE
COORDINATOR
801 533-6161

Utah Department of Health
Family Health Services Division
Salt Lake City 84113

*SALT LAKE CITY
Intermountain Regional
Poison Control Center
50 N. Medical Drive
84132
801 581-2151

VERMONT

STATE
COORDINATOR
802 862-5701

Department of Health
Burlington 05401

BURLINGTON
Vermont Poison Center
Medical Center Hospital
05401
802 658-3456

VIRGINIA

STATE
COORDINATOR
804 786-5188

Bureau of Emergency Medical Services
Richmond 23219

ALEXANDRIA
Alexandria Hospital
4320 Seminary Rd.
22314
703 370-9000   Ext. 555

ARLINGTON
Arlington Hospital
5129 N. 16th St. 22205
703 558-6161

BLACKSBURG
Montgomery County
Community Hosp.
Rt. 460, S. 24060
804 951-1111

CHARLOTTESVILLE
Blue Ridge Poison Center
University of Virginia
Hospital 22908
804 924-5543

*AAPCC Designated Regional Center

DANVILLE
Danville Memorial Hosp.
142 S. Main St.
22201
804 799-2100   Ext. 3869

FALLS CHURCH
Fairfax Hospital
3300 Gallows Rd.
22046
703 698-3600
698-3111

HAMPTON
Hampton General Hosp.
3120 Victoria Blvd. 23661
804 722-1131

HARRISONBURG
Rockingham Memorial Hosp.
738 S. Mason St.
22801
804 434-4421   Ext. 225

LEXINGTON
Stonewall Jackson Hosp.
22043
804 463-9141

LYNCHBURG
Lynchburg Gen. Marshall
Lodge Hosp., Inc.
Tate Springs Rd. 24504
804 528-2066

NASSAWADOX
Northampton-Accomack
Memorial Hosp. 23413
804 442-8000

NORFOLK
DePaul Hospital
Granby St. at Kingsley
Lane 23505
804 489-5111

PETERSBURG
Petersburg General Hosp.
801 South Adams St. 23803
804 861-2992

PORTSMOUTH
U.S. Naval Hospital
23708
804 397-6541   Ext. 418

RICHMOND
Virginia Poison Center
Virginia Commonwealth Univ.
Box 763 MCV Station 23298
804 786-9123

ROANOKE
Roanoke Memorial Hosp.
Belleview at Jefferson St.
P.O. Box 13367 24033
703 981-7336

STAUNTON
King's Daughters' Hosp.
P.O. Box 2007
24401
703 885-0361   Ext. 209, 247

WAYNESBORO
Waynesboro Community
Hospital
501 Oak Ave. 22980
703 942-8355   Ext. 440, 500

WILLIAMSBURG
Williamsburg Community
Hospital
Mt. Vernon Ave.
Drawer H 23185
804 229-1120   Ext. 65

VIRGIN ISLANDS

STATE
COORDINATOR
809 774-1321
Ext. 275

Department of Health
St. Thomas 00801

ST. CROIX
Charles Harwood Memorial
Hospital
Christiansted
00820
809 773-1212
773-1311 Ext. 221

Ingeborg Nesbitt Clinic
Fredericksted 00840
809 772-0260
772-0212

ST. JOHN
Morris F. DeCastro Clinic
Cruz Bay 00830
809 776-1468

ST. THOMAS
Knud-Hansen Memorial
Hospital
00801
809 774-1321 Ext. 224, 225

WASHINGTON

STATE
COORDINATOR
206 522-7478

Department of Social & Health Services
Seattle 98115

ABERDEEN
St. Joseph's Hospital
1006 North H St.
98520
206 533-0450 Ext. 277

BELLINGHAM
St. Luke's General Hosp.
809 E. Chestnut St.
98225
206 676-8400
676-8401
1-800 562-8816
562-8817
(TOLL FREE)

LONGVIEW
St. John's Hospital
1614 E. Kessler
98632
206 636-5252

MADIGAN
Madigan Army Medical
Ctr. Emergency Rm.
98431
206 967-6972

OLYMPIA
St. Peter's Hospital
413 N. Lilly Rd.
98506
206 491-0222

*AAPCC Designated Regional Center

*SEATTLE
Children's Orthopedic
Hosp. & Med. Ctr.
4800 Sandpoint Way, N.E.
98105
206 634-5252

SPOKANE
Deaconess Hospital
W. 800 5th Ave.
99210
509 747-1077

TACOMA
Mary Bridge Children's
Hospital
311 S. L St. 98405
206 272-1281   Ext. 259

VANCOUVER
St. Joseph Community
Hospital
600 N.E. 92nd St.
98664
206 256-2067

YAKIMA
Yakima Valley Memorial
Hospital
2811 Tieton Dr. 98902
509 248-4400

WEST VIRGINIA

STATE
COORDINATOR
304 348-2971

Department of Health
Charleston 25305

CHARLESTON
West Virginia Poison
System
3110 McCorkle Avenue SE
25304
304 348-4211

MORGANTOWN
Mountain State Poison Ctr.
Department of Pediatrics
West Virginia University
Medical Center 26506
304 293-5341

WISCONSIN

STATE
CONTACT
608 267-7174

Department of Health & Social Services, Div. of Health
Madison 53701

EAU CLAIRE
Luther Hospital
1225 Whipple
54701
715 835-1515

GREEN BAY
St. Vincent Hospital
835 S. Van Buren St.
54305
414 433-8100

*AAPCC Designated Regional Center

LACROSSE
St. Francis Hospital
700 West Avenue, N.
54601
608 784-3971

MADISON
University Hospitals &
Clinics
600 Highland Avenue
53792
608 262-3702

MILWAUKEE
Milwaukee Children's
Hospital
1700 W. Wisconsin
53233
414 931-4114

WYOMING

STATE
COORDINATOR
307 777-7955

Office of Emergency Medical Services
Department of Health & Social Services
Cheyenne 82001

CHEYENNE
Wyoming Poison Center
DePaul Hospital
2600 East 18th St.
82001
307 635-9256

Appendix II

List of Selected Abbreviations

ACS	American Chemical Society
BRH	Bureau of Radiological Health
CCERP	DHHS Committee to Coordinate Environmental and Related Programs
CDC	Center for Disease Control
CEC	Commission of the European Communities
CEQ	Council on Environmental Quality
CHEMRIC	Chemical Monograph Referral Center
CHRIS	Chemical Hazard Response Information Center
CIIT	Chemical Industry Institute of Toxicology
CIS	Centre International d'Informations de Securite [International Occupational Safety and Health Information Centre]
CMA	Chemical Manufacturers Association
CPSC	Consumer Product Safety Commission
CSIN	Chemical Substances Information Network
CTFA	Cosmetic, Toiletry and Fragrance Association
DHHS	Department of Health and Human Services [formerly DHEW]
DOE	Department of Energy
DOT	Department of Transportation
ECDIN	Environmental Chemicals Data and Information Network
EDF	Environmental Defense Fund
EEC	European Economic Community

EIC	Environmental Information Center
EMIC	Environmental Mutagen Information Center
EPA	Environmental Protection Agency
ETIC	Environmental Teratogen Information Center
FAO	Food and Agricultural Organization
FDA	Food and Drug Administration
FIFRA	Federal Insecticide, Fungicide, and Rodenticide Act
FSQS	Food Safety and Quality Service [of the USDA]
GEMS	Global Environmental Monitoring System
IARC	International Agency for Research on Cancer
ICGEC	Interagency Collaborative Group on Environmental Carcinogenesis
ILO	International Labour Organization
IRCC	Information Response to Chemical Crisis
IRLG	Interagency Regulatory Liason Group
IRPTC	International Register of Potentially Toxic Chemicals
IRRC	Interagency Radiation Research Council
ITSDC	Interagency Toxic Substances Data Committee
NCI	National Cancer Institute
NCTR	National Center for Toxicological Research
NEISS	National Electronic Injury Surveillance System
NEPA	National Environmental Policy Act
NIEHS	National Institute of Environmental Health Sciences
NIOSH	National Institute for Occupational Safety and Health
NLM	National Library of Medicine
NOAA	National Oceanic and Atomspheric Administration
NPCN	National Poison Center Network
NRC	Nuclear Regulatory Commission
NTP	National Toxicology Program
OECD	Organization for Economic Cooperation and Development
OSHA	Occupational Safety and Health Administration
PMA	Pharmaceutical Manufacturers Association
RCRA	Resource Conservation and Recovery Act
SIS	Specialized Information Services Division [of the NLM]
SOT	Society of Toxicology
TIP	Toxicology Information Program

Appendix II: List of Selected Abbreviations

TIRC	Toxicology Information Response Center
TIS	Toxicology Information Subcommittee [of the ITSDC]
TOSCA	Toxic Substances Control Act
TSSC	Toxic Substances Strategy Committee
UNEP	United Nations Environment Programme
USDA	United States Department of Agriculture
WHO	World Health Organization

Appendix III

Additional Information Resources

These late arrivals consist of items recently published, forthcoming, or otherwise relevant and not included in the main body of this work. Elsevier has kindly agreed to add on this addendum very close to press time in order to provide as much up-to-date material as possible. A simplistic and intuitive risk assessment was performed by the author, who concluded that the benefit of providing the reader with these additional items would outweigh the risk of potential confusion that this separate listing might precipitate. It is the responsibility of us all to continue the relentless pursuit of the toxicology literature.

BOOKS

Analytical Toxicology

1558. Baselt RC. *Biological Monitoring Methods for Industrial Chemicals.* Davis, CA. Biomedical Publications. 1980.

> Presents data on a wide range of chemicals with significant industrial exposures. Information on occurrence, blood concentrations, metabolism and excretion, toxicity, biological monitoring and a variety of analytical methods such as gas chromatography, colorimetry, and spectrometry.

1559. Schuetzle D, ed. *Monitoring Toxic Substances.* Washington, DC. American Chemical Society. 1979.

> Volume 94 of the ACS Symposium Series. Techniques such as atomic absorption spectrometry, inductively coupled plasma-atomic emission spectroscopy, surface microanalytical methods, Fourier transform infrared analysis, and opto-acoustic spectroscopy are covered.

Carcinogenesis, Mutagenesis, Teratogenesis

1560. Demopoulos HB, Mehlman MA, eds. *Cancer and the environment: an academic review of the environmental determinants of cancer relevant to prevention.* Park Forest South, IL. Pathotox. 1980.

A diverse group of papers from a symposium held in cooperation with the American Cancer Society. Some subject areas were inhibitors of carcinogens, DNA damage, mammalian cell transformation, promotion and cofactors, epidemiology, multiple factors, the "urban factor," hair dye components, lipids, free radical reactions, steroids, nutrient deficiencies, endogenous nitrite formation in man, saccharin, cyclamates, drugs, and occupational cancer.

1561. Felkner IC, ed. *Microbial testers: probing carcinogenesis.* New York. Marcel Dekker. 1981.

Volume 5 of the *Microbiology Series.* Provides information on the use of short-term bacterial assays.

1562. Juchau MR, ed. *The biochemical basis of chemical teratogenesis.* New York, Elsevier/North-Holland. 1981.

Focuses on the biochemical means by which chemicals produce dysmorphogenic effects.

1563. Kimmel CA, Buelke-Sam J, eds. *Developmental toxicity.* New York. Raven Press. 1981.

Covers development and differentiation, developmental determinants of toxicity, perinatal and postnatal functional evaluations, and assessment of test methodology.

1564. Neubert D, Merker HJ, Nau H, Langman J, eds. *Role of pharmacokinetics in prenatal and perinatal toxicology.* Stuttgart. Thieme. 1978.

Papers from a symposium which discussed "problems concerning the significance of drug metabolism in fetal and neonatal tissues, of placental passage and of other factors . . ."

1565. Nicholson WJ, ed. *Management of Assessed Risk for Carcinogens.* New York. New York Academy of Sciences. 1981.

1566. Rice JM. *Transplacental Carcinogenesis.* New York. Raven Press. 1981.

1567. Sax NI, Weisburger E. *Cancer Causing Chemicals.* New York. Van Nostrand Rheinhold. 1981.

1568. Sontag JM, ed. *Carcinogens in Industry and the Environment.* New York. Marcel Dekker. 1981.

Volume 16 of the *Pollution Engineering and Technology Series*. Papers on workplace carcinogens, in vitro screening, carcinogens in food and plants, cosmetics, ionizing radiation, etc.

1569. Walters DB, ed. *Safe Handling of Chemical Carcinogens, Mutagens, Teratogens and Highly Toxic Substances,* 2 volumes. Ann Arbor, MI. Ann Arbor Science. 1980.

"The emphasis of this book is on the control and use of hazardous agents in a research organization." Sections on laboratory design and management, chemical monitoring and medical surveillance, informational needs, structure-activity relationships, spill control, and disposal.

See also:

Costa M. *Metal Carcinogenesis Testing.* [under *Metals*]

Gustafsson J. *Biochemistry, Biophysics and Regulation of Cytochrome P-450.* [under *Miscellaneous*]

Vainio H. *Occupational Cancer and Carcinogenesis.* [under *Occupational Health and Industrial Hygiene*]

Cosmetics

See also:

Cronin E. *Contact Dermatitis.* [under *Target Systems*]

Gloxhuber C. *Anionic Surfactants.* [under *Environmental Toxicology*]

Drugs

1570. Gram TE, ed. *Extrahepatic Metabolism of Drugs and Other Foreign Compounds.* New York. SP Medical. 1980.

Volume 5 of *Monographs in Pharmacology and Physiology*. Reviews metabolism in sites such as the kidney, lung, placenta, small intestine, gonads, eyes and skin. In addition, despite the title, there is a major review on drug metabolism in the liver.

1571. de Gruchy GC. *Drug-induced Blood Disorders.* Oxford. Blackwell Scientific Publications. 1975.

"The aim of this book is to present an account of haematological reactions which may occur as the result of the administration of drugs."

1572. Grundmann E, ed. *Drug-induced Pathology.* New York. Springer-Verlag. 1980.

Volume 69 of *Current Topics in Pathology*. Includes contributions on epidemiology, pathophysiology, cancer, drug-induced liver disease, drug-induced kidney disease, and prenatal toxicology.

See also:

Neubert D. *Role of Pharmacokinetics in Prenatal and Perinatal Toxicology.* [under *Carcinogenesis, Mutagenesis, Teratogenesis*]

Environmental Toxicology

1573. Bitton G, Damron BL, Edds GT, Davidson JM, eds. *Sludge—Health Risks of Land Application.* Ann Arbor, MI. Ann Arbor Science. 1980.

This volume represents "an assessment of the state-of-the-art regarding the health risks associated with the use of sewage sludge in a soil-plant-animal food production system."

1574. Brown RC, Chamberlain M, Davies R, Gormley IP, eds. *The In Vitro Effects of Mineral Dusts.* London. Academic Press. 1980.

Broad subject areas covered in this book—in vitro reactivity of mineral dusts, macrophages, dust-biological membrane interactions, chemical modifications, welding fumes, primary cell and organ culture, and inflammatory response and fibrosis.

1575. Cowser KE, ed. *Synthetic Fossil Fuel Technology: Potential Health and Environmental Effects.* Ann Arbor, MI. Ann Arbor Science. 1980.

Topics such as chemical characterization, biological effects, environmental transport, and occupational health control technology are treated.

1576. Eaton JG, Parrish PR, Hendricks AC, eds. *Aquatic Toxicology.* Philadelphia. American Society for Testing Materials. 1980.

Proceedings of the Third Annual Symposium on Aquatic Toxicology held in New Orleans in 1978. Papers grouped into the broad headings of "Toxicology Methods Development," "Bioconcentration: Water Quality Management," "Effluent Testing," and "Physiology and Behavior: Single Toxicant Effects."

1577. Gloxhuber C, ed. *Anionic Surfactants: Biochemistry, Toxicology, Dermatology.* New York. Marcel Dekker. 1980.

"The research findings compiled for this monograph on toxicological and dermatological properties and on the amounts absorbed by man are of great practical importance for the calculation of health risks in a great variety of applications, for instance in the fields of detergents and cosmetics.'' Includes acute, subacute, and chronic toxicity data, a large chapter on local tolerance in animal tests, dermatologic observations in humans, and studies on carcinogenic, mutagenic, and teratogenic properties.

1578. Griest WG, Guering MR, Coffin DL. *Health Effects Investigation of Oil Shale Development.* Woburn, MA. Ann Arbor Science. 1981.

Investigates potential health effects in production and refining of shale oil.

1579. Grosjean D, ed. *Nitrogenous Air Pollutants: Chemical and Biological Implications.* Ann Arbor, MI. Ann Arbor Science. 1979.

Explores health effects and chemical reactions of nitrogenous pollutants such as nitrogen oxides, peroxynitric acid, ammonia, amines, etc.

1580. Lee SD, Mudd JB, eds. *Assessing Toxic Effects of Environmental Pollutants.* Ann Arbor, MI. Ann Arbor Science. 1979.

Discusses methods useful in assessing toxicity and determining underlying mechanisms.

1581. McKinney JD, ed. *Environmental Health Chemistry: The Chemistry of Environmental Agents as Potential Human Hazards.* Ann Arbor, MI. Ann Arbor Science. 1981.

After an introductory section of papers on environmental health chemistry, the book is divided into sections on environmental analysis, structure-activity and toxicity prediction, and chemistry aspects of toxicological testing.

1582. National Research Council. *Drinking Water and Health,* 3 volumes. 2-3. Washington, DC. National Academy Press. 1980.

1583. Rom WN, Archer VE, eds. *Health Implications of New Energy Technologies.* Woburn, MA. Ann Arbor Science. 1980.

Analyzes new technologies such as coal-conversion, oil shale retorting, and geothermal energy. Discusses health problems and risks.

1584. Sittig M, ed. *Priority Toxic Pollutants: Health Impacts and Allowable Limits.* Park Ridge, NJ. Noyes Data. 1980.

''A practical manual of priority toxic pollutants arranged alphabetically in encyclopedic form . . . explicit, instant information for the characterization and identification, as well as the allowable levels of 65 priority toxic pollutants, their derivatives or degradation products or intermedia transfers.'' Includes data such as toxic effects, current levels of exposure, special groups at risk, existing guidelines and standards, EPA criteria summations, and basis for proposed human health criteria.

1585. Trieff NM, ed. *Environment and Health.* Ann Arbor, MI. Ann Arbor Science. 1980.

Current information on health effects of air pollutants, water pollutants, heavy metals, water re-use, noise, and other topics.

1586. Wadden RA, ed. *Energy Utilization and Environmental Health: Methods for Prediction and Evaluation of Impact on Human Health.* New York. Wiley. 1978.

Considers public health effects in the planning and use of energy production technologies. Chapters on hypersusceptible populations, body burdens, pollutant dispersal in air and water, etc.

1587. Weber LJ, ed. *Aquatic Toxicology,* volume 1. New York. Raven Press. 1981.

Reviews toxicity data in aquatic organisms and compares these with higher vertebrate data.

1588. Willeke K, ed. *Generation of Aerosols and Facilities for Exposure Experiments.* Ann Arbor, MI. Ann Arbor Science. 1980.

Although more related to instrumentation and facilities than specific health effects, this volume has been included because of man's widespread exposure to aerosols and the importance of accurate exposure experiments. Section I covers basic concepts of aerosol generation and health effects. Section II focuses on methods of aerosol generation. Section III covers exposure facilities utilizing models for man and animals.

See also:

Calabrese EJ. *Nutrition and environmental health.* [under *Food*]

Demopoulos HB. *Cancer and the environment.* [under *Carcinogenesis, Mutagenesis, Teratogenesis*]

Food

1589. Graham HD, ed. *The safety of Foods,* 2nd ed. Westport, CT. AVI Publishing. 1980.

This multiauthored text ranges over the spectrum of food safety issues. Papers on food poisoning, mycotoxins, nitrosamines, mercury, PCBs, pesticide residues, irradiated foods, toxins in plants, food additives, toxins in plants, etc.

1590. Calabrese EJ. *Nutrition and Environmental Health: The Influence of Nutritional Status on Pollutant Toxicity and Carcinogenicity,* 2 volumes. New York. John Wiley. 1980.

Critically assesses nutritional status as a factor in the etiology of toxicity and carcinogenicity. Volume 1 focuses on the vitamins while volume 2 concentrates on minerals and macronutrients.

1591. Lueck E. *Antimicrobial Food Additives.* Berlin. Springer-Verlag. 1980.

An enlarged and revised translation of *Chemische Lebensmittelkonservierung,* published in 1977. Introductory chapters on general topics of analysis, health aspects, legal status, antimicrobial action. Remaining chapters deal with different preservatives. Synonyms, history, properties, production, regulatory status, antimicrobial action, and fields of use are discussed with substantial space devoted to health aspects, including LD50s and other toxicity data.

1592. Somogyi JC, Tarjan R, eds. *Foreign Substances and Nutrition.* Basel. Karger. 1980.

Number 29 of *Bibliotheca Nutritio et Dieta.* Papers on pesticides in food, nitrites, sweetening agents, lead and cadmium, naturally occurring toxicants, etc.

1593. Vettorazzi G. *Handbook of International Food Regulatory Toxicology.* Jamaica, NY. Spectrum. 1980.

1594. Wurtman RJ, Wurtman JJ, eds. *Toxic Effects of Food Constituents on the Brain.* New York. Raven Press. 1979.

Volume 4 of the series *Nutrition and the Brain.* Reviews such areas as hyperkinesis, glutamic acid neurotoxicity, and roles of peptides.

Metals

1595. Costa M. *Metal Carcinogenesis Testing: Principles and In Vitro Methods.* Clifton, NJ. Humana Press. 1980.

"... explains fundamental principles of metal carcinogenesis as they are currently understood, and provides detailed practical descriptions of rapid and inexpensive in vitro assay methodology presently in use for the detection of potentially carcinogenic metals and their compounds."

1596. Nriagu JO, ed. *The Biogeochemistry of Mercury in the Environment.* Amsterdam. Elsevier/North-Holland. 1979.

Volume 3 of *Topics in Environmental Health.* "... a comprehensive

review and assessment of the sources, mechanisms of transport, trans-
formations and sinks of mercury in the environment, as well as the
effects of mercury in animals, humans, vegetation and the aquatic
biota.''

1597. Nriagu J, ed. *Cadmium in the Environment.* New York. John Wiley.
1980.

Part 1 concentrates on ecological cycling while part 2 discusses health
effects.

1598. Nriagu J, ed. *Copper in the Environment.* New York. John Wiley. 1980.

Part 1 concentrates on ecological cycling while part 2 discusses health
effects, including environmental and occupational exposures.

1599. Nriagu JO, ed. *Nickel in the Environment.* New York. John Wiley.
1980.

''... deals comprehensively with the sources, distribution, behavior
and flow of nickel in different ecosystems; it also delves into the
metabolism, biochemistry, and systemic toxicity of nickel in plants,
human beings, and other organisms... carcinogenic and dermatological effects of nickel and with the interactions of nickel with essential
minerals.''

1600. Nriagu J, ed. *Zinc in the Environment.* New York. John Wiley. 1980.

Part 1 concentrates on ecological cycling while part 2 discusses health
effects.

Occupational Health and Industrial Hygiene

1601. Anderson KE, Scott RM. *Fundamentals of Industrial Toxicology.*
Woburn, MA. Ann Arbor Science. 1981.

A compact reference to the essential aspects of industrial toxicology.

1602. Schilling RSF. *Occupational Health Practice,* 2nd ed. London. Butterworth. 1981.

Provides information on occupational health practices in different parts
of the world. ''New material on the effects of work exposures on organ
systems, screening of organ systems, toxicity testing, occupational
health in developing countries, and the health of migrant workers is
included in this 2nd edition.''

1603. Vainio H, Sorsa M, Hemminki K, eds. *Occupational Cancer and Carcinogenesis.* Washington. Hemisphere Publishing. 1981.

An historical perspective on occupational cancer is followed by sections on etiology, molecular carcinogenesis, detection, epidemiology, risk, and risk assessment. Some of the industries considered in the papers are PVC, plastics, foundries, and rubber. Even includes a chapter on "the morals of risk assessment."

See also:
Baselt RC. *Biological Monitoring Methods for Industrial Chemicals.* [under *Analytical Toxicology*]

Physical Hazards

1604. Casarett GW. *Radiation Histopathology,* 2 volumes. Boca Raton, FL. CRC Press. 1981.

Concentrates on ionizing radiation in mammalian organs.

1605. Harm W. *Biological Effects of Ultraviolet Radiation.* Cambridge. Cambridge University Press. 1980.

1606. Hubner KF, Fry SA, eds. *The Medical Basis for Radiation Accident Preparedness.* New York. Elsevier North Holland. 1980.

Covers total body irradiation, acute local irritation, medical response to acute radiation exposure, role of cytogenetics in biological dosimetry, long term effects, and reactor accidents.

1607. Illinger KH, ed. *Biological Effects of Ionizing Radiation.* Washington. American Chemical Society. 1981.

1608. Tobias JV, Jansen G, Ward WD, eds. *Noise as a Public Health Hazard.* Rockville, MD. American Speech-Language-Hearing Association. 1980.

Papers in such areas as noise-induced hearing loss, nonauditory physiological effects, influence on behavior, community response, interactions between noise and other physical/chemical agents. A substantial compendium.

See also:
Gilbert HA. *Radiation damage to the nervous system.* [under *Target Systems*]

Target Systems

1609. Chubb IW, Geffen LB, eds. *Neurotoxins: Fundamental and Clinical Advances.* Adelaide, Australia. Adelaide University Press. 1979.

Emphasizes reptile, marine, and chemical neurotoxins.

1610. Cronin E. *Contact Dermatitis.* Edinburgh. Churchill Livingstone. 1980.

"An account of the clinical features of allergic contact dermatitis . . . for practising dermatologists in an endeavor to make patch
testing more comprehensible and encourage greater use of this investigation." Among the substances covered are clothing and textiles,
cosmetics, foods, drugs, metals, pesticides, plants, woods, photosen-
sitizers, plastics, preservatives, and rubber. An excellent source for
effects of agents on the skin.

1611. Hook JB, ed. *Toxicology of the Kidney.* New York. Raven Press. 1981.

Discusses chemically induced injury to the kidney.

1612. Merigan W, Weiss B, eds. *Neurotoxicity of the Visual System.* New
York. Raven Press. 1980.

Includes substances related to fossil fuel technologies, methylmercury,
and various common contaminants and their effects on the visual system.

1613. Mitchell CL, ed. *Nervous System Toxicology.* New York. Raven Press.
1981.

"Discusses the behavioral, neurophysiological, neurochemical, and
morphological aspects of nervous system toxicology, and assesses the
predictiveness and limitations of test methods currently used."

1614. Plaa GL, Hewitt WR, eds. *Liver Toxicity.* New York. Raven Press. 1981.

1615. Prasad KN, Vernadakis A, eds. *Mechanisms of Neurotoxin Substances.*
New York. Raven Press. 1981.

Molecular, cellular, and organismic effects on nervous tissue are discussed.

1616. Sanders CL, ed. *Pulmonary Toxicology of Respirable Particles.* Oak
Ridge, TN. Technical Information Center, U.S. Department of Energy.
1980.

1617. van Stee EW, ed. *Cardiovascular Toxicology.* New York. Raven Press.
1981.

A review of the cardiovascular system is followed by sections on animal studies and cell culture technology relevant to the system. Finally,
the toxicodynamics of different classes of chemicals and natural substances are discussed.

1618. Witschi H, Nettesheim P, eds. *Mechanisms in Respiratory Toxicology*. Boca Raton, FL. CRC Press. 1981.

See also:

Gram TE. *Extrahepatic Metabolism of Drugs and Other Foreign Compounds*. [under *Drugs*]

de Gruchy GC. *Drug-induced Blood Disorders*. [under *Drugs*]

Wurtman RJ. *Toxic Effects of Food Constituents on the Brain*. [under *Food*]

Miscellaneous

1619. Bierlein LW. *Red Book on Transportation of Hazardous Materials*. Boston. CBI Publishing. 1977.

1620. Bretherick L. *The Handbook of Reactive Chemical Hazards,* 2nd ed. Woburn MA. Butterworths. 1979.

> Over 7000 entries with data on stabilities, violent interactions, fire information. Structural formulas provided.

1621. Cooney DO. *Activated Charcoal: Antidotal and Other Medical Uses*. New York. Marcel Dekker. 1980.

> Covers in vivo adsorption and adsorption studies involving viruses, bacteria, vitamins, hormones, toxins, etc.

1622. Gustafsson J, Carlstedt-Duke J, Mode A, Rafter J, eds. *Biochemistry, Biophysics and Regulation of Cytochrome P-450*. Amsterdam. Elsevier/North-Holland. 1980.

> Papers on the chemical characterization, mechanisms of regulation, mechanism of action, molecular biology, and biophysical characterization of cytochrome P-450 as well as a section on cytochrome P-450 and steroids. "The interest in cytochrome P-450 has been especially stimulated as a consequence of the ongoing shift of emphasis within basic cancer research towards chemical carcinogenesis, where cytochrome P-450 mediated metabolic activation of precarcinogens is an important issue."

1623. Hayes AW, ed. *Methods in Toxicology*. New York. Raven Press. 1981.

> Concentrates on testing methods in toxicology, including those used to comply with regulatory standards. Specific organ systems discussed.

1624. McCann M, Barazani M, eds. *Health Hazards in the Arts and Crafts.* Washington, DC. Society for Occupational and Environmental Health. 1980.

Fascinating papers on hazards associated with such activities as jewelry making, performing arts, stained glass, sculpting, potting, etc. Includes case studies, research in workplace monitoring, evaluation of ingredients, and a substantial section devoted to regulatory and legal issues.

1625. Pojasek RB, ed. *Toxic and Hazardous Waste Disposal,* 6 volumes. Woburn, MA. Ann Arbor Science. 1979–1981.

Not directly concerned with health effects but a valuable supplementary reference that fully covers the topic of dangerous wastes.

1626. Reeves AL, ed. *Toxicology: Principles and Practice.* Volume 1. New York. John Wiley. 1981.

Papers on the basics of toxicology, including metabolism, sensory irritation, mutagenesis, cancer, etc. Derived from papers presented at Wayne State University's short course entitled "Principles and Practice of Industrial Toxicology."

1627. Tu AT, ed. *Survey of Contemporary Toxicology.* Volume 1. New York. John Wiley. 1980.

Provides an overview of the following areas: industrial toxicology, chemical water pollutants, food additives, foodborne diseases, bacterial toxins, plant toxins, and marine toxins.

PERIODICALS

1628. *American Journal of Industrial Medicine.* New York. Alan R. Liss. 1, 1980–

The inaugural issue featured articles in such areas as asbestos disease among ship repair workers, mental symptoms in lacquerers, solvent poisoning, flight attendants' exposure to ozone, a mortality study of newspaper printing workers and brain cancer in petrochemical workers.

1629. *Art Hazards Newsletter.* New York. Center for Occupational Hazards.

1630. *Dangerous Properties of Industrial Materials Report.* New York. Van Nostrand Reinhold. 1, 1980–

Each issue begins with a few feature articles and is followed by data on hazardous materials. Information on these materials includes CAS and NISOH identifying numbers, synonyms, uses, toxicity data, environmental impact, information on storage and handling, recent Federal

Register citations, selected structural formulas, references, and other sources of information. Editor-in-chief is N. Irving Sax and this is a fine updating source to his *Dangerous Properties of Industrial Materials.*

1631. *Recent Advances in Occupational Health.* Edinburgh. Churchill Livingstone. 1981–

1632. *Risk Analysis.* New York. Plenum. 1, 1981–

The official journal of the Society of Risk Analysis. "Will cover topics of great interest to regulators, researchers, and scientific administrators. It will deal with health risks and thus will involve workers in cancer research, medical genetics, mutagenesis, epidemiology, teratology and toxicology . . . engineering risks . . . mathematical and theoretical aspects . . . social and psychological aspects."

1633. *Xenobiotica.* London. Taylor & Francis. 1, 1971–

Papers concentrate on the metabolic transformation of exogenous chemicals in biological systems.

AUDIOVISUALS

1634. *Lectures in Toxicology*
(Slides)
Zbinden G, ed
Oxford. Pergamon Press. 1980–1981.

This new series of lectures consists of 35 mm color and monochrome slides with presentation notes. It has been exclusively designed for toxicology and pharmacology teachers. Each lecture is written by specialists in the field and is devoted to a specific subject. Available in English, French, Spanish, German, and Japanese. The first eight lectures are:

1. Histopathology of experimental toxic neuropathies
2. Effect of contraceptive steroids on mammary tumor development in beagles.
3. Test systems in mutagenicity: in vitro cytogenetics.
4. Oxygen-induced lung damage: 1—the chemistry of oxygen reduction.
5. Oxygen-induced lung damage: 2—pulmonary oxygen toxicity.
6. Drug-induced retinopathy: 1—causal and clinical aspects.
7. Drug-induced retinopathy: 2—pathogenesis and experimental pathology.
8. Toxicologic implications of drug-induced peroxisome proliferation.

ORGANIZATIONS

1635. *American Conference of Governmental Industrial Hygienists*
P.O. Box 1937
Cincinnati, OH 45201

A professional society whose membership consists of governmental employees involved in industrial hygiene.

1636. *American Occupational Medical Association*
150 N. Wacker Drive
Chicago, IL 60606

Members are primarily physicians specializing in occupational medicine. Provides continuing education, conducts scientific meetings. Publishes *Journal of Occupational Medicine*.

1637. *Center for Occupational Hazards*
Five Beekman Street
New York, NY 10038

Concentrates on collecting and disseminating information on health hazards associated with arts and crafts. Operates the Art Hazards Information Center and publishes *Art Hazards Newsletter*.

1638. *Coalition for Health and the Environment*
1500 Wilson Boulevard
Suite 807
Arlington, VA 22209

Membership consists of some 180 industry, labor, insurance, health professional, consumer, and environmental groups. The coalition promotes disease prevention to policymakers, private industry, and the public.

1639. *International Union of Toxicology (IUTOX)*
Dr. Robert G. Burford/Secretary-General, IUTOX
c/o G. D. Searle & Co. of Canada, Ltd.
400 Iroquois Shore Road
Oakville, Ontario, Canada L6H 1M5

Established during the Second International Congress on Toxicology held in Brussels in July 1980. The Union will foster international cooperation in the science of toxicology and sponsor future congresses in the field. Various international, national, and regional organizations devoted to toxicology and related disciplines will be invited to join.

1640. *National Research Council of Canada*
Ottawa, Canada K1A OR6

Considerable and significant toxicological work is being performed by this agency, particularly its Associate Committee on Scientific Criteria for Environmental Quality. They have published numerous substantive reviews on substances such as ethylenethiourea, mercury, asbestos, sulfur, noise, and arsenic. For information on the activities of this committee contact the Environmental Secretariat at the above address.

1641. *Society of Environmental Toxicology and Chemistry*
P.O. Box 352
Rockville, MD 20850

Incorporated in November 1979 as a professional society concerned with the impact of chemicals and technology on the environment. Multidisciplinary approaches utilizing chemical, physical, and biological data are sought. Promotes research, education, and training. The second annual meeting is scheduled for November 1981 in Washington. Arrangements are being made for the publication of a professional journal.

1642. *Society for Occupational and Environmental Health*
1341 G Street, NW
Washington, DC 20005

A professional association concerned with occupational and environmental health issues. Sponsors workshops and conferences. Recently published *Health Hazards in the Arts and Crafts*.

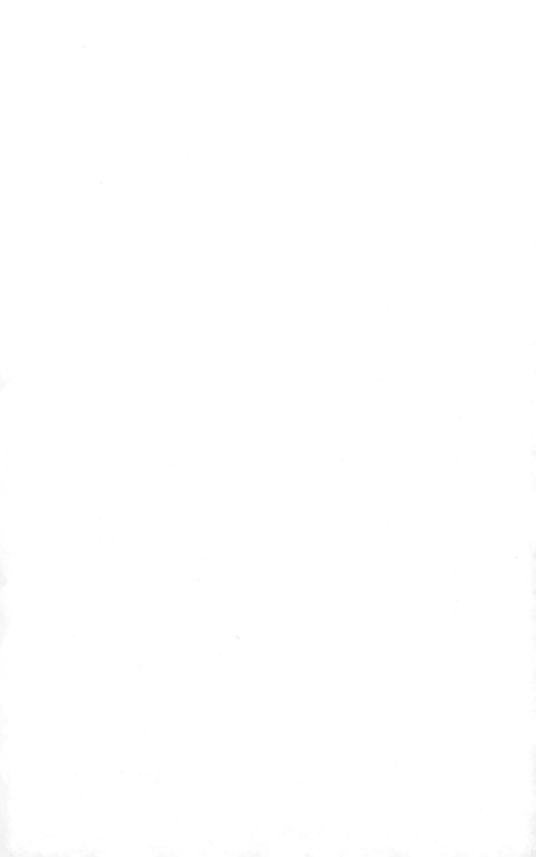

Subject Index

Numbers refer to entry numbers, not page numbers.

298

Mycotoxins [cont.]
Uraguchi, K., Yamazaki, M. *Toxicology, Biochemistry, and Pathology of Mycotoxins*, 30

N

Nasopharyngeal Carcinoma
IARC Scientific Publication. *Nasopharyngeal Carcinoma: Etiology and Control*, 334
National Institute of Environmental Health Sciences (NIEHS), Annual Report
Schambra, P.E. *Federal agency support for environmental health research: A report by the National Institute of Environmental Health Sciences*, 366
National Toxicology Program (NTP), Annual Report
Review of current DHEW research related to toxicology, and *Annual Report*, 367
Naturally Occurring Substances
IARC Monograph. *Some Naturally Occurring Substances*, 299
Neurotoxicology
Lectures in Toxicology, 1634
Manzo, L. *Advances in Neurotoxicology*, 251
Mitchel, C.L. *Nervous System Toxicology*, 1616
Spencer, P.S., Schaumburg, M.D. *Experimental and Clinical Neurotoxicology*, 258
Vinken, P.J., Bruyn, G.W. *Intoxications of the Nervous System*, 261
Neurotoxicology of the Eye
Merigen, W., Weiss, B. *Neurotoxicity of the Visual System*, 1615
Neurotoxicology, Radiation-Induced
Gilbert, H.A., Kagan, A.R. *Radiation Damage to the Nervous System: A Delayed Therapeutic Hazard*, 248
Neurotoxins
Chubb, I.W., Geffen, L.B. *Neurotoxins: Fundamental and Clinical Advances*, 1612
Neurotoxins, Mechanisms
Prasad, K.N., Vernadakis, A. *Mechanisms of Neurotoxin Substances*, 1618
Nickel
IARC Monograph. *Cadmium, Nickel, Some Epoxides, Miscellaneous Industrial Chemicals, and General Considerations on Volatile Anaesthetics*, 300
National Research Council. *Nickel*, 356
Nriagu, J.O. *Nickel in the Environment*, 1602

Nitrofurans
Carcinogenesis: A Comprehensive Survey, 419
IARC Monograph. *Some Anti-Thyroid and Related Substances, Nitrofurans and Related Substances, Nitrofurans and Industrial Chemicals*, 296
Nitrogen Oxides
Environmental Health Criteria. *Oxides of Nitrogen*, 364
Lee, S.D. *Nitrogen Oxides and Their Effects on Health*, 129
National Research Council. *Nitrogen Oxides*, 357
Nitrosamines, Volatile, Analysis
IARC Scientific Publication. *Environmental Carcinogens—Selected Methods of Analysis. Volume 1: Analysis of Volatile Nitrosamines in Food*, 332
N-Nitroso Compounds
Environmental Health Criteria. *Nitrates, Nitrites, and N-Nitroso Compounds*, 364
IARC Monograph. *Some Aromatic Amines, Hydrazine and Related Substances, N-Nitroso Compounds and Miscellaneous Alkylating Agents*, 293
IARC Monograph. *Some Inorganic Substances, Chlorinated Hydrocarbons, Aromatic Amines, N-Nitroso Compounds, and Natural Products*, 290
IARC Monograph. *Some N-Nitroso Compounds*, 306
IARC Scientific Publication. *Environmental Aspects of N-Nitroso Compounds*, 333
IARC Scientific Publication. *Environmental N-Nitroso Compounds—Analysis and Formation*, 328
IARC Scientific Publication. *N-Nitroso Compounds Analysis and Formation*, 317
IARC Scientific Publication. *N-Nitroso Compounds in the Environment*, 323
Noise
Environmental Health Criteria. *Noise*, 364
Henderson, D., et al. *Effects of Noise on Hearing*, 230
May, D.N. *Handbook of Noise Assessment*, 231
Noise and hearing loss, 544
Olishifski, P.E., Harford, E.R. *Industrial Noise and Hearing Conservation*, 237
Tobias, J.V., et al. *Noise as a Public Health Hazard*, 1611
Nutrition
Calabrese, E.J. *Nutrition and Environmental*

Journal Article Index

Numbers refer to entry numbers, not page numbers.

Miller, R.W. Environmental causes of cancer in childhood, 1545

Trosko, J.E., Chang, C.C. Environmental carcinogenesis: an integrative model, 1117

Carcinogenesis, In Vitro

DePaolo, J.A., Castro, B.C. In vitro carcinogenesis with cells in early passage, 967

Carcinogenesis, and Mutagenesis

Troski, J.E., Chang, C.C. Relationship between mutagenesis and carcinogenesis, 1119

Carcinogenesis Screening

Purchase, I.F. Procedures for screening chemicals for carcinogenicity, 1070

Carcinogens

Hoffman, D., Wynder, E.L. Identification and reduction of carcinogens in the respiratory environment, 1009

McGarity, T.O. Substantive and procedural discretion in administrative resolution of science policy questions-regulating carcinogens in EPA and OSHA, 1354

Melzer, M.S. Paradox of carcinogens as cell destroyers and cell stimulators. A biochemical hypothesis, 1029

Merrill, R.A. Regulating carcinogens in food: legislators guide to the food safety provisions of the Federal Food, Drug, and Cosmetic Act, 1357

Montesano, R. The use of mutagenicity tests in screening chemical carcinogens, 1040

Nagao, M. et al. Environmental mutagens and carcinogens, 1046

Poirier, L.A., Weisburger, E.K. Selection of carcinogens and related compounds tested for mutagenic activity, 1065

Cell Cycle Mutants

Simchen, G. Cell cycle mutants, 1092

Cell Lines

Zachowski, A., et al. Cell lines with altered membrane structures for comprehensive studies of cancer cells, 1141

Cereal Grains

Lorenz, K. Ergot on cereal grains, 894

Cervicobrachial Syndromes, Occupational

Waris, P. Occupational cervicobrachial syndromes: a review, 1452

Chemical Dumps

Koch, K. Seeping from under the carpet: Cleaning up chemical dumps posing dilemma for Congress, 1343

Chemical Hazards

McLean, A.E. Hazards from chemicals:

scientific questions and conflicts of interest, 1355

Chemical Spills

Croke, K.G., Raufer, R.K. Management of toxic chemical spills, 1325

Chemicals, Dietary

Sub-threshold levels of dietary chemicals and mixed function oxidase induction, 1501

Chemicals, Occupational

Hemminki, et al. Genetic risks caused by occupational chemicals. Use of experimental methods and occupational risk group monitoring in the detection of environmental chemicals causing mutations, cancer and malformations, 1000, 1432

Chemosterilants

Labrecque, G.C., Fye, R.L. Cytogenetic and other effects of the chemosterilants tepa, metepa, apholate and hempa in insects: a review, 1481

Chlordane

Chlordane, 953, 1462

Chloroform

Chloroform, 954

Chloroprene

Haley, T.J. Chloroprene (2-chloro-1, 3-butadiene)—what is the evidence for its carcinogenicity?, 993

Chocolate

Fries, J.H. Chocolate: a review of published reports of allergic and other deleterious effects, real or presumed, 1293

Cholera Toxin

Neckers, L.M. Cholera toxin action in the central nervous system: effects on serotonin metabolism, 904

Chromosome Aberrations

Grant, W.F. Chromosome aberrations in plants as a monitoring system, 1260

Chrysotherapy

Gibbons, R.B. Complications of chrysotherapy: a review of recent studies, 1393

Ciliates

Persoone, G., Dive, D. Toxicity tests on ciliates: a short review, 1272

Cinnamic Aldehyde

Mathias, C.G., et al. Contact urticaria from cinnamic aldehyde, 1177

Cinnamyl Anthranilate

Cinnamyl anthranilate, 1152

Circadian Rhythms

Aschoff, J. Features of circadian rhythms relevant for the design of shift schedules, 1422

315

329